Psychiatry's Contract with Society
Concepts, controversies, and consequences

Psychiatry's Contract with Society
Concepts, controversies, and consequences

FIRST EDITION

Edited by

Dinesh Bhugra
Amit Malik
George Ikkos

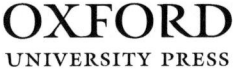

OXFORD
UNIVERSITY PRESS

Great Clarendon Street, Oxford OX2 6DP

Oxford University Press is a department of the University of Oxford.
It furthers the University's objective of excellence in research, scholarship,
and education by publishing worldwide in

Oxford New York

Auckland Cape Town Dar es Salaam Hong Kong Karachi
Kuala Lumpur Madrid Melbourne Mexico City Nairobi
New Delhi Shanghai Taipei Toronto

With offices in

Argentina Austria Brazil Chile Czech Republic France Greece
Guatemala Hungary Italy Japan Poland Portugal Singapore
South Korea Switzerland Thailand Turkey Ukraine Vietnam

Oxford is a registered trade mark of Oxford University Press
in the UK and in certain other countries

Published in the United States
by Oxford University Press Inc., New York

© Oxford University Press, 2011

The moral rights of the author have been asserted
Database right Oxford University Press (maker)

First published 2011

All rights reserved. No part of this publication may be reproduced,
stored in a retrieval system, or transmitted, in any form or by any means,
without the prior permission in writing of Oxford University Press,
or as expressly permitted by law, or under terms agreed with the appropriate
reprographics rights organization. Enquiries concerning reproduction
outside the scope of the above should be sent to the Rights Department,
Oxford University Press, at the address above

You must not circulate this book in any other binding or cover
and you must impose the same condition on any acquirer

British Library Cataloguing in Publication Data
Data available

Library of Congress Cataloging in Publication Data
Data available

Typeset in Minion by Glyph International Bangalore, India
Printed in Great Britain
on acid-free paper by
CPI Antony Rowe, Chippenham, Wiltshire

ISBN 978–0–19–9566778

10 9 8 7 6 5 4 3 2 1

Oxford University Press makes no representation, express or implied, that the drug
dosages in this book are correct. Readers must therefore always check the product
information and clinical procedures with the most up-to-date published product
information and data sheets provided by the manufacturers and the most recent codes of
conduct and safety regulations. The authors and the publishers do not accept responsibility
or legal liability for any errors in the text or for the misuse or misapplication of material in
this work. Except where otherwise stated, drug dosages and recommendations are for the
non-pregnant adult who is not breastfeeding.

Preface

Dinesh Bhugra, Amit Malik, and George Ikkos

An emphasis on public good, both of patients and of the population at large, is part of the responsibility of the psychiatrist. With changes in the scientific basis of psychiatry and an increased accessibility of knowledge, not only are the patient and carer expectations changing but also those of society at large. Increasing levels of consumerism and commodification of medicine mean that the power equation between the clinician and the patient is becoming more balanced. Patient expectations of the therapeutic encounter have changed. Society expects physicians and psychiatrists to be caring, well trained, to keep up to date, and provide care that will at least not be intentionally harmful to the patient. In return, doctors—including psychiatrists—expect society to treat them with respect and trust, and to provide financial rewards and social status that are appropriate and commensurate with their skills. Such a contract has never been explicit but is implicit. With the medical scandals that have occurred in the last quarter of a century in the United Kingdom and the United States, it has become necessary to review this contract, and this volume is an attempt to do just that. There is also the need to be more introspective and to examine our own skills, contributions, and moral values. Unprompted by external influences, we need to take time to assess, and if necessary, revise our core values of professionalism and our relationship with society.

The concept of the contract is implicit and relies heavily on the concepts of professionalism. It focuses on the relationship between peers, patients and clinicians, and society and clinicians, and this is the basis of what the practice of medicine and psychiatry is about. Working with other professions, patients, and carers as well as other stakeholders is a crucial part of the function of the psychiatrist. Society expects psychiatrists to provide clinical leadership in service planning and service delivery. Broad-based training and learning about professional values and attributes makes psychiatrists indispensable in providing clinical leadership and working with partners in a sensible manner. The old paternalistic style of delivering medical care has already given way to a more collaborative joint working with patients and their carers. Thus, acknowledging patient autonomy and constantly striving to provide high quality evidence-based treatments is at the heart of professionalism. A major responsibility of the psychiatrist is to advocate for patients, their needs, and services in the face of ever-increasing alienation and stigmatizing attitudes of society. Therefore, psychiatrists need to work with members of society to educate and support each other. Social attitudes will influence psychiatric care and psychiatrists must take these into account. This contract with society is crucial for psychiatry and psychiatrists, and it must be reviewed regularly.

The contributors to this volume are truly international in their status, scope, and knowledge. We are thankful that they agreed to contribute to this book and that they met the due deadlines. It made the entire project valuable and eminently enjoyable. Martin Baum and his production team at OUP have been hugely supportive without being intrusive, and we acknowledge their support. Andrea Livingstone provided sterling assistance, and her organization skills, keen attention to detail, and unflinching patience made the editors' task that much easier. Our grateful thanks.

Contents

Preface *v*
Contributors *ix*

1 Introduction *1*
   Dinesh Bhugra
2 Psychiatry, professionalism, and society: a note on past and present *9*
   George Ikkos
3 Professions, related occupations, and ethics *23*
   Robin Downie
4 What is expected of doctors? *35*
   Lord Victor Adebowale
5 Economics and society: efficiency, equity, and choice *43*
   Paul Freddolino and Martin Knapp
6 Stakeholders' expectations of psychiatric professionalism *59*
   Dinesh Bhugra, Susham Gupta, Genevieve Smyth, and Martin Webber
7 Training and professionalism *73*
   Greg Lydall and Amit Malik
8 Psychiatry's contract with society: what do clinical psychiatrists expect? *89*
   Daniel McQueen, George Ikkos, Paul St John-Smith, Philip Kemp, Povl Munk-Jørgensen, and Albert Michael
9 Teaching professionalism *103*
   Richard L. Cruess and Sylvia R. Cruess
10 Medicine's social contract with society: its nature, evolution, and present state *123*
    Sylvia R. Cruess and Richard L. Cruess
11 The role of psychiatrists and their professional associations in the regulation and performance management of mental health services *147*
    Paul Lelliott
12 Professionalism, regulation, scrutiny, and litigation *163*
    Carole Kaplan
13 Psychiatry's contract with society: a personal perspective from England *171*
    Hugh Griffiths

14 Psychiatry's contract with society: revalidation and professionalism *181*
Laurence Mynors-Wallis

15 Professionalism and medicine: a managerial perspective *195*
Naaz Coker

16 Changing professionalism *209*
Edwin Borman

17 Psychiatric ethics and the 'new professionalism' *221*
Michael Robertson and Garry Walter

18 Psychiatry's contract: where next? *241*
Dinesh Bhugra and Amit Malik

Index *245*

Contributors

Lord Victor Adebowale
The House of Lords
London, UK

Dinesh Bhugra
Professor of Mental Health &
Cultural Diversity
Institute of Psychiatry, King's College
London, UK

Edwin Borman
Consultant Anaesthetist
University Hospitals Coventry &
Warwick
Coventry, UK

Naaz Coker
Chair, St George's Healthcare
NHS Trust
St George's Hospital
London, UK

Richard Cruess
Professor of Orthopedic Surgery
Centre for Medical Education
McGill University
Montreal, Quebec
Canada

Sylvia Cruess
Professor of Medicine
Centre for Medical Education
McGill University
Montreal, Quebec
Canada

Robin Downie
Emeritus Professor of Moral Philosophy
Glasgow University
Glasgow, UK

Paul Freddolino
Professor of Social Work,
Michigan State University
East Lansing, Michigan, USA, and
Visiting Senior Fellow,
London School of Economics
London, UK

Hugh Griffiths
Deputy National Clinical Director
for Mental Health
Department of Health
London, UK

Susham Gupta
Consultant Psychiatrist
East London NHS Foundation Trust
Assertive Outreach Team - City &
Hackney
London, UK

George Ikkos
Consultant Psychiatrist & Director of
Medical Education
Barnet Enfield & Haringey Mental
Health NHS Trust
London, UK

Carole Kaplan
Associate Medical Director
Children & Young People's Services
Northumberland, Tyne & Wear
NHS Trust
Newcastle, UK

Philip Kemp
Director of Health Studies
University of East London
London, UK

Martin Knapp
Professor of Health Economics and Director, Centre for the Economics of Mental Health
Institute of Psychiatry
King's College London, and
Professor of Social Policy and Director of Personal Social Services Research Unit
London School of Economics
London, UK

Paul Lelliott
Director, College Centre for Quality Improvement
Royal College of Psychiatrists
London, UK

Greg Lydall
Specialty Trainee in Psychiatry and Honorary Researcher
University College London
London, UK

Daniel McQueen
Consultant Adolescent Psychiatrist
Barnet Enfield and Haringey Mental Health NHS Trust
London, UK

Amit Malik
Associate Medical Director
Consultant Psychiatrist in Old Age Psychiatry
Phoenix Day Hospital
Gosport War Memorial Hospital
Gosport
Hampshire, UK

Albert Michael
Consultant Psychiatrist in Adult Psychiatry & Director of Medical Education
Suffolk Mental Health Partnership Trust
UK

Povl Munk-Jørgensen
Professor of Psychiatry, Aarhus University
Chief Consultant, Research Director & Head of Unit for Psychiatric Research
Aalborg Psychiatric Hospital
University Hospital
Aarhus, Denmark

Laurence Mynors-Wallis
Consultant Psychiatrist and Medical Director
Dorset Healthcare NHS Foundation Trust
Bournemouth, UK

Michael Robertson
Senior Staff Specialist Psychiatrist,
Sydney South West Area Health Service
Clinical Senior Lecturer, Discipline of Psychological Medicine, and Senior Lecturer, Centre for Values, Ethics and the Law in Medicine,
University of Sydney
Sydney, Australia

Paul St John-Smith
Consultant Community Psychiatrist
Hertfordshire Partnership Foundation NHS Trust (Mental Health)
UK

Genevieve Smyth
Professional Affairs Officer for Mental Health and Learning Disabilities
College of Occupational Therapists
London, UK

Garry Walter
Professor of Child and Adolescent Psychiatry, Discipline of Psychological Medicine, University of Sydney
Area Clinical Director, Child and Adolescent Mental Health Services
Northern Sydney Central Coast Health
Sydney, Australia

Martin Webber
Programme Leader & Learning and
Teaching Coordinator
Institute of Psychiatry
King's College London
London, UK

Chapter 1

Introduction

Dinesh Bhugra

Health care delivery is decided by the society at large and health care professionals work within the political, social, and economic contexts. These contexts can change and clinical practice therefore changes accordingly. The relationship between the professionals as care givers and the society is a complex one. Professionals deliver the care from within the society and are also members of the society who contribute to the functioning of the society through a number of sources. This relationship (between the clinician and society) undoubtedly affects the therapeutic encounter between the patient and the clinician, which lies at the heart of any health care delivery.

Code of conduct

Professionalism and its codes of conduct have been in the public domain for centuries, and society has been a part of this discussion either directly or indirectly. Present day coda of ethics have emerged as a result of an implicit contract with society. There is a historical aspect to this that illustrates the role of the state in developing and controlling the codes of practice.

Sox (2007) points out that codes of professional conduct are tangible expressions of professionalism. Medieval guilds controlled entry into a craft, setting standards for training and quality. The State set to control these in the cause of the spread of capitalism, as they were seen to be monopolistic providers. Something similar is beginning to emerge now in the United Kingdom with pressures on the medical profession and in increasing control in a number of ways. This may reflect a gradual spread of capitalism into the NHS with increased privatization of services and supportive components of the service. From 1100 to 1500 AD, as the guilds became the organizing principles for skilled work, they controlled the opportunities for training through restricting entry into the guilds, options of types of training, available number of apprentice placements, controlling the machinery, and the rates of production. Guilds and their monopolistic positions were seen as a threat to capitalism (see Krause, 1996 for details). The power of guilds lost to strong central government initiated controls in Western Europe at slightly difference paces. For example, France and England seemed to be ahead compared with Italy and Germany, which may be because of different social and political factors. Krause (1996) defines the State as bodies that possess a monopoly over the means of force as well as most of the means of sustaining the society. These include education and professional training. Capitalism is a political economic system that focuses on individual owners or shareholders making profit. When the guilds were being challenged, it was their monopoly position. Again, in a similar way, the medical profession as a monopoly health care provider is under threat because the group is being seen as monopolistic, and other professions, such as nurses and psychologists, are being allowed to prescribe drugs, albeit still limited in some countries.

Society's dissatisfaction with the medical profession can be related to increased bureaucracy, limited access to services, increased demands irrespective of need, along with a number of changes in the society and society's expectation of the medical profession. Zuger (2004) notes that the twentieth century professionalism within medicine was clear – pride, accomplishment, and authority –and by the mid-twentieth century these values provided loyal patients, respectful colleagues, job security, good social and economic status. In the United States, with increasing costs and improved technical knowledge, demands increased. In addition, increased levels of management by insurance companies and other providers and of litigiousness meant that external factors made professionals feel besieged. Internal factors such as an increasing workload meant reduced time for family, friends, or leisure with increased work-related stress, reduced income, and prestige. Zuger (2004) suggests that causes of dissatisfaction also included increased administration, increased number of patients, limitations on drug prescriptions, insurance stipulations, and reduced personal well-being among others. Holsinger and Beaton (2006) note that physicians have struggled to keep their individualism.

Society and the contract with psychiatry

The contract between psychiatry and its practitioners on the one hand and the society at large on the other is an implicit one and not an explicit one. Cruess (2006) suggests that medicine's relationship with society has been seen as a contract, which has inbuilt obligations and expectations on the part both of the society and the profession. She noted that the idea of the social contract emerged 300 years or so earlier when society granted the profession monopoly over the knowledge base, autonomy in practice and associated (professional and secondarily social and economic) status and rewards, along with the privilege of self-regulation. These components of the contract were based on the assurances from the profession that in return the profession will ensure professional competence, probity, integrity, and high moral standards of its members. As Cruess (2006) points out, in the nineteenth century and up to the middle of the twentieth century, society believed that the medical profession was not abusing its position of monopoly and was maintaining acceptable standards. However, this changed dramatically in both the United States and the United Kingdom. With increasing costs and medical scandals, there was a general feeling often encouraged by the politicians that the medical profession was not to be trusted. In the United Kingdom various enquiries into scandals challenged directly or indirectly the notions of self-regulation. Changing public expectations, increasing demands, and crumbling services (in the United Kingdom at least) meant that public confidence in the profession's ability to self-regulate and maintain standards was shaken very badly.

Medicine as a profession also became a major industry and the shift towards perceived self-interest and self-promotion by physicians contributed to lowering of prestige and status. With an increase in numbers of medical schools opening with very limited control of standards meant that society started seeing the profession as self-serving. More than 70 years ago, Gough (1936) had observed that the rights and duties of the state and its citizens are reciprocal, and this reciprocity (and its recognition by both sides) constitutes a relationship which by analogy can be called a social contract. The contract is based on mutual expectations and obligations between health care professionals and society. Cruess (2006) pointed out that society expects that medicine will provide services of a healer who is competent, moral, accountable, and transparent. In addition, such an individual is able to provide objective advice and altruistic service. Probity and honesty in all the links are of significance here. In return, Cruess (2006) argues that medicine expects society to trust the profession, allow it autonomy and self-regulation. Medicine also expects the health care system to be adequately funded and value-driven and allow it to participate in public policy and have a shared responsibility (between society and medicine) for health. There is also an expectation that medicine can run as a monopoly and provide financial and non-financial (i.e. status) rewards. In a number of ways these expectations are real but therein also lies a series of problems. The contract is unwritten; however the ethics and the codes applicable to the profession are not. This means that public or societal expectations can change suddenly in response to scandals – real or imagined - and a knee-jerk response may challenge any of the underlying assumptions and expectations. As the social contract is unwritten, the mutual hostility may put extra pressure on both sides. The contract keeps evolving as a result of changes in social expectations, health care system and its funding, and other factors such as the development of new therapeutic interventions and specialisms in the profession. Cruess (2006) suggests that, irrespective of different health care systems, expectations of society and doctors of each other remain broadly similar. Altruism and its definitions may well change because in privately funded systems what is understood by altruism may well be different than in a wholly publicly funded health care system. Expecting doctors to be healers and competent in what they do also depends upon how they are trained and how this training is funded. The notions of self-regulation may be shifting from 'self' as in a collective professional self of the group to an individual 'self'.

Threats to professionalism

Doctors' dissatisfaction with society reflects a broader degree of disillusionment because they feel that either the society is becoming too interfering or is not offering expected levels of support and not meeting some of its own obligations. If an implicit contract exists then negotiating the details of the contract becomes a legitimate professional activity. To provide good acceptable services the profession of medicine should develop services that will be influenced by the human and economic resources available. Patients and society share responsibility for health; clinicians also form a part of the society and their contributions also influence policy, thereby making the contract a complex one (see Figure 1.1).

The role of autonomy, while being a part of the society, complicates matters further. Although a hallmark of the profession and granted sufficient freedom,

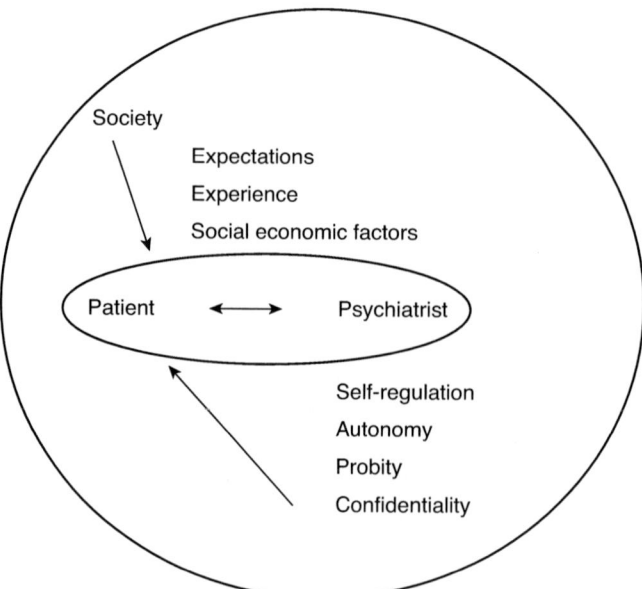

Fig. 1.1 Interaction between society and medicine

autonomy is never unlimited (Cruess, 2006) and this often gets ignored by the profession that may like unfettered autonomy.

The psychiatrist under this implicit contract has multiple levels of responsibility from personal to the patient, professional (to the profession he or she belongs), and societal (to the larger society). Sometimes these levels may be in conflict with each other but the ultimate responsibility is to the patient, who must remain at the centre of clinical practice. Patients deserve to be treated in a holistic manner, taking into account their physical, spiritual, and mental needs. Furthermore, it is the society that defines sickness and deviance thereby encouraging the profession to develop new categories of diagnosis or abandon the old ones. Understanding patient needs in the context of their family, culture, and society and understanding societal expectations are important concepts within the rubric of professionalism.

Evidence-based psychiatry

A major challenge for psychiatry is that it is perceived anti-scientific even though it is not entirely true. There are clinical practice guidelines developed and used in several countries and these are based on evidence currently available even if it does not give the full picture. A distrust of the system on the part of the psychiatrist and a distrust of psychiatry on the part of patients and their carers can lead to misunderstanding of each other's perspectives, and prejudice and fear become more rampant on the patient's side. This stigma needs to be taken on board by the psychiatrist to ensure that patients and their carers see services as emotionally accessible. Explanatory models used by patients and their carers must be taken into account and used as part of the dialogue between the patient and the psychiatrist and between the psychiatrist and society. If the patient's explanatory models are totally at odds with that of the rest of the society the reasons and possible explanations for that need to be understood. Psychiatrists have the skills to incorporate a number of complex aetiological factors to develop intervention strategies. Using the resources available through other professionals in the team, the psychiatrist can build suitable support systems and treatment strategies. Psychiatry as a specialty deals with both mind and brain and the relationships between mentally ill individuals and the society at large. Using principles of health economics it appears that psychiatrists need to be clear about the difference between output and outcome. The challenge is whether treatment A works better than treatment B and which of the two is cost-effective. This is where clinical practice guidelines come in. These strategies indicate clear goals of care and highlight potentially beneficial therapeutic approaches (O'Connor, 2005). In addition, these may reduce variations in care and post code lottery. However, they may not work for comorbid conditions and may not work for all conditions and not for all patients. It is treating the patient in a holistic manner which is of paramount importance. Treatment guidelines are evidence-based but also focus on short-term conditions (Tinetti, Bogardus, & Agostini, 2004). Benefit/harm ratio and patient preferences may also influence the usefulness of clinical practice guidelines.

Patient-based psychiatry

There is no doubt that medicine in general and psychiatry in particular have the patient at the core of the therapeutic encounter. Patient-based psychiatry also indicates that patients and their carers can become advocates for psychiatry and psychiatrists in the same way that psychiatrists are advocates for their patients and the profession. Patient-based psychiatry relies on the view by the psychiatrist that as a healer and clinician, the reduction in distress is the key. Skills required are learnt over a period of training and gaining experience both through direct clinical care and knowledge. Roter and Hall (2004) point out that patient centredness is among the key indicators for future quality of health care agenda. Patient centredness is not only a philosophy of medicine but also has professional and moral imperatives. Within this interaction are contents related to the communication style and quality of care indicators (Roter & Hall, 2004). There are differences between male and female physicians in that both groups use different styles for communication and data gathering. In addition to communication, mindful clinical practice includes active observation of oneself (on the part of the clinician), the patient, and the problem; critical curiosity, pre-attention processing; willingness to examine and set aside categories and prejudices; humility to tolerate awareness of one's area of incompetence and compassion based on insight (Epstein, 1999). Equally, patients are more likely to disclose their problems depending upon a number of factors. Disclosure of psychosocial information by the patient was noted to be strongly associated with questions being asked about psychosocial factors (Wissow, Roter, & Wilson, 1994).

Conclusion

The contract between the profession of psychiatry and society is implicit but mutual understanding of positions from which each side is coming and an agreement on the way forward is crucial. The profession needs to respond to changing demands and expectations from the patients and their carers and, equally, patients and their carers need to be aware of newer treatments and interventions and focus on need rather than demand.

This volume is an attempt to bring together experts in the field, clinicians, managers, health economists, and other stakeholders to open up a discussion on the next steps for psychiatry's contract with society.

References

Cruess, S. R. (2006). Professionalism and medicine's social contract with society. *Clinical Orthopaedics and Related Research,* **449**,170–176.

Epstein, R. M. (1999). Mindful practice. *JAMA,* **282**, 833–839.

Gough, J. W. (1936). *The Social Contract: A Critical Study of Its Development.* Oxford: Clarendon Press.

Holsinger, J. W., & Beaton, B. (2006). Physician professionalism for a new century. *Clinical Anatomy,* **19**, 473–479.

Krause, E. A. (1996). *Death of the Guilds.* New Haven, CT: Yale University Press.

O'Connor, P. J. (2005). Adding value to evidence based clinical guidelines. *JAMA,* **294**, 741–743.

Roter, D. L., & Hall, J. A. (2004). Physician gender and patient centred communication: A critical review of empirical research. *Annual Review of Public Health,* **25**, 497–519.

Sox, H. (2007). The ethical foundations of professionalism: a sociologic history. *Chest,* **131**, 1532–1540.

Tinetti, M. E., Bogardus, S. T., & Agostini, J. V. (2004). Potential pitfalls of disease-specific guidelines for patients with multiple conditions. *NEJM,* **351**, 2870–2874.

Wissow, L. S., Roter, D. L., & Wilson, M. E. H. (1994). Paediatrician interview style and mothers: disclosure of psychosocial issues. *Paediatrics,* **93**, 289–295.

Zuger, A. (2004). Dissatisfaction with medical practice. *NEJM,* **350**, 69–75.

Chapter 2

Psychiatry, professionalism, and society: a note on past and present

George Ikkos

Introduction

The International Labour Organisation Standard Classification of Occupations (2008) defines doctors as those who 'diagnose and treat human physical and mental illnesses, disorders, and injuries, and recommend preventive action based on the scientific principles of modern medicine. They may specialize in certain disease categories or methods of treatment, or assume responsibility for the provision of continuing and comprehensive medical care to individuals, families, and communities'.

Johann Christian Reil, Professor of Medicine in Halle, Germany, first used the term psychiatry in 1808 (Marneros, 2008). He emphasized the inseparability of physical and mental, the importance of psychosomatics and psychotherapy, and the need to develop a psychology that addresses the specific reality of people with mental disorder. Henry Miller, a neurologist and friend of psychiatrists, wrote in 1997 that the psychiatrist '… must be first and foremost and all the time a physician. In fact, psychiatry is neurology without physical signs, and calls for diagnostic virtuosity of the highest order. The simple fact is that a psychiatrist is a physician who takes a proper history at the first consultation' (quoted in Craddock et al., 2008).

In 'Good Psychiatric Practice' The Royal College of Psychiatrists (2009) noted, under the heading 'Core attributes':

> Patients, their carers, their families and the public need good psychiatrists. Good psychiatrists make the care of their patients their first concern: they are competent; keep their knowledge up to date; are able and willing to use new research evidence to inform practice; establish and maintain good relationships with patients, carers, families and colleagues; are honest and trustworthy, and act with integrity. Good psychiatrists have good communication skills, respect for others and are sensitive to the views of their patients, carers and families.

An ideal early psychiatrist was the late eighteenth century French physician Philippe Pinel (Appignanessi, 2008, chapter 2). Pinel was appointed in 1793 the first medical head of Bicetre Hospice in post-revolutionary France and was later awarded the first chair of hygiene in the newly formed Ecole de Medicine de Paris. In 1795 he was appointed professor of pathology and transferred to Salpetriere. He translated William Cullen's *First Lines in the Treatment of Physik* and three volumes of the *Philosophical Transactions* of the Royal Society. In 1798 he published his *Nosologie Philosophique* in which he combined his detailed clinical observations (in conformity with the then prevalent method of *la clinique* in France) with John Locke's theories on the association of ideas. It is an early example of cognitive approaches to psychopathology.

Pinel famously took the chains off his patients and advocated *la douceur* (a winning gentleness) in approaching them. He also advocated (1) psychodrama for treatment of delusions, (2) placing patients with 'invented families' for rehabilitation, and (3) the hiring of convalescent patients as nurses. In such proposals he anticipated by 200 years modern proposals such as 'recovery' and 'social inclusion' (Care Services Improvement Partnership et al., 2007; Royal College of Psychiatrists Social Inclusion Scoping Group, 2009) and properly ensured the breadth of the role of the psychiatrist against any narrow interpretation of Miller's observations (see above).

It is the combination of deep commitment to humanity and healing, clinical observation and practice, and scholarship and public mental health that makes Pinel such an outstanding example of professionalism in psychiatry. Since Pinel's time enormous progress has been made both in the sciences basic to psychiatry (biology, psychology, sociology, anthropology, epidemiology, etc) and their practical application in various assessment and treatment modalities (social, psychological, and biological) (Gelder, Andreasen, Lopez-Ibor Jr, & Geddes, 2009; Tyrer & Silk, 2008). The lay reader may find accessible information on the fruits of progress in the 'mental health information' pages of the website of the Royal College of Psychiatrists (www.rcpsych.ac.uk).

Early development and failure of the modern profession

In Pinel's work, excellence in psychiatry is found before the term itself was coined. Doctors have been treating mental illness since earliest antiquity (Porter R, 2002, chapters 1–3). Specialist wards for the mentally ill could be found in hospitals in the Arab world as early as the eighth century CE. There are known cases of officially recognized senior clinicians examining junior practitioners in Baghdad, Iraq in the tenth and eleventh centuries, and Damascus, Syria, in the eleventh century (Pormann & Savage-Smith, 2007, chapter 3). The competence of medical practitioners wishing to earn admitting rights in hospitals at the time, including the mental health wards had to be assessed by their peers.

Perhaps the earliest specialist institution for the mentally ill in Europe was St Mary Bethlehem, London in the thirteenth century (surviving today as the Bethlem Royal Hospital). Early asylums under religious authority were also established in fifteenth century in Spain in the cities of Valencia, Zaragoza, Seville, Valladolid, Toledo, and Barcelona (Porter R, 2002, chapter 5). Private institutions specializing in the care of the mentally ill also flourished from around the same time (Jones, 2002, chapters 1–2, Porter R, 2002, chapters 4–5).

In England the College of Physicians, London was granted Royal charter by King Henry VIII in 1515. The duties of the few members of the highly prestigious Royal College have included the oversight of the quality of care received by patients in private 'madhouses' in London, in particular those placed by local parishes at public expense. It was the failure of the Royal College of Physicians in London and private medical and other proprietors in the provinces to ensure humane standards of care as well as the appalling conditions of the mentally living in poorhouses and workhouses during the time of the Industrial Revolution in the United Kingdom, that led to a wave of legislation, beginning in the late eighteenth century and continuing actively in the next that helped establish the extensive network of public mental asylums in this country in the nineteenth and early twentieth centuries (Jones, 1993, chapters 2–5). Only after law and public authorities established the mental asylums the profession of psychiatry began to form (Bewley, 2008). The Association of Medical Officers of Asylums for the Insane (later the Medicopsychological Association, then the Royal Medicopsychological Association and now the Royal College of Psychiatrists) was formed in 1841. Similarly the Association of Superintendents of American Institutions for the Insane, later to become the American Psychiatric Association, was formed in 1844 (Musto, 2009). The teaching of psychiatry in medical schools was first introduced in the United Kingdom in the University of London only in 1865.

Whereas in the United Kingdom and United States psychiatry emerged out of the asylums, in Germany, it emerged out of universities (Porter R, 1997, chapter 16). Nineteenth century German academic psychiatrists such as Alzheimer, Kraepelin, and Wernicke were pioneers in describing psychiatric syndromes and investigating their links with the brain. Higgins and George (2007) summarized with remarkable clarity the progress in the 'neuroscience of clinical psychiatry' since then.

The creation of professional associations of psychiatrists and research and teaching of the subject in medical schools has not always been an effective guarantee for quality of services. For example, in the United Kingdom public mental health services had attracted such opprobrium by the late 1960s and early 1970s that the then minister of health, Keith Joseph (later Sir Keith Joseph), played an active part in establishing the Royal College of Psychiatrists in 1972. It was part of an effort to improve standards of services and particularly standards of training of doctors working in them (Rivett, 2006, chapter 3).

The most spectacular failure of the profession to protect the mentally ill and learning disabled occurred in Nazi Germany in the middle of twentieth century. Paediatricians, inspired by nowadays notorious notions of 'life unworthy of life' and beginning in Leipzig in 1933, had actively engaged in killing severely disabled children in paediatric hospital wards by using lethal injections. They were followed in the 1940s by German asylum doctors who certified adult mentally ill, learning disabled, and epileptic patients as 'unworthy of life'. This led to the extermination of approximately 100,000 such patients, initially by injection and later in gas chambers (Friedlander, 1995, chapters 1–3).

Six German psychiatric 'hospitals' (Grafeneck, Brandenburg, Harteheim, Sonnesnstein, Brenburg, and Hadamar) served as a grotesque vanguard for the later extension of killing to other German citizens, especially Jews, and eventually many others from beyond (Friedlander, 1995, chapters 4–6). Max de Crinis, Werner Heyde, Berthold Kihn, Friedrich Mauz, Friedrich Panse, Kurt Polisch, Carl Schneider, and Werner Willinger, all professors of psychiatry, were involved in these Nazi crimes (Friedlander, 1995).

Professionalism, psychiatry, and society

Kuczewski (2006) defined professionalism in medicine as 'the norms that guide the relationships in which physicians engage in the care of patients'. Musto (2009) highlighted Dr Thomas Percival's publication of a formal statement on medical ethics in 1803 as an early modern example of attempts to clarify in detail expectations of physicians' actual conduct in hospitals rather than simply expressing more abstract ideals. The document arose out of disputes between doctors who had visiting rights to the Manchester Infirmary. Although not writing exclusively for psychiatrists, Percival does address the treatment of mentally ill patients, as they were included in the population of the infirmary along with others. Percival wrote as follows (quoted in Musto, 2007, p. 13):

> The law justifies the beating of a lunatic, in such a manner as the circumstances may require. But it has been before remarked that a physician, who attends an asylum for insanity, is under an obligation of honour as well as of humanity to secure to the unhappy sufferer, committed to his charge, all the tenderness and indulgence compatible with steady and effectual government. And the strait wastecoat [sic], with other improvements in modern practice, now preclude the necessity of coercion by corporal practice.

The statement of Percival reminds us that abusive treatment has been espoused as good treatment. The treatment of King George III in eighteenth century England in the hands of Dr Willis (not a physician!) is another example, which confirms that the otherwise privileged and rich mentally ill shared in the fate of those even less fortunate in this respect (Jones, 1993).

The Royal College of Physicians (London) (RCP) (2005) defined professionalism as 'a set of values, behaviours and relationships that underpins the public trust in doctors'. The RCP adds that the purpose of medicine is realized through 'a partnership between patient and doctor, based on mutual respect, individual responsibility and appropriate accountability'.

Mental health service users have an important role in defining professionalism and combating stigma and abuse. An early example of an influential service user is Clifford Beers, a Yale graduate and Boston businessman (Porter R, 2002, chapter 7). His book on *The Mind that Found Itself* (1908) is a classic. As a young man he was hospitalized from 1901 to 1903 in (1) Stamford Hall, (2) Hartford Retreat, and (3) Connecticut Hospital for the Insane – two private and one public mental health institutions in the United States. He was treated with the straitjacket and punitive cruelty. He stated, 'My attendants were incapable of understanding the operations of my mind, and what they could, they could not tolerate.' After recovery he cooperated with psychologists such as William James and doctors such as Silas Weir Mitchell to set up the Mental Hygiene Movement. The movement survives as 'Mental Health America' (www.mentalhealthamerica.net) and its members sit on the board of major mental health organizations in that country.

Modern notions of partnership between physician/psychiatrist and patient/service user have a history therefore (Rose & Lucas, 2007). The same applies for the non-professional carers and families of the mentally ill (Magliano, McDaid, Kirkwood, & Berzins, 2007). The Mental Aftercare Association, an organization of non-professional carers in the United Kingdom, which has endured and is now called 'Together' (www.together-uk.org) was formed towards the end of the nineteenth century (Jones, 1993, chapter 7). Mental health services users and carers are having increasing input in the training of psychiatrists (Ikkos, 2003, 2005; Yousif, 2009).

Professionalism implies a contract between the medical profession and society (Bhugra, 2008). Poverty and social exclusion, although not essential or unique to mental illness, undoubtedly add to the plight of the mentally ill and, indeed, sometimes bring forward such plight (Royal College of Psychiatrists Social Inclusion Scoping Group, 2009). Politicians have an important role in negotiating and supporting professionalism.

An outstanding early example of an important politician for psychiatry is the seventh Earl of Shaftsbury in the United Kingdom (Jones, 2002, chapters 3 and 4).

He entered the House of Commons as Lord Ashley and joined a select committee to consider the state of pauper lunatics in 1828. He was instrumental over a whole parliamentary career in advancing legislation that created the system of public mental health asylums in the United Kingdom. Today we tend to think of these as places of social exclusion but at the time they were the product of genuine concern about the welfare of the mentally ill and the risks of abuse and exploitation in the community and in poorhouses and workhouses. It was 'community psychiatry' in this sense. Roy Porter's (2002, pp. 117–118) quote from Dr A.W.F. Brown in 1837, head of an asylum in Montrose, Scotland conveys the idealism that some politicians and doctors shared at the time:

> Conceive a spacious building resembling the palace of a peer, airy and elevated, and elegant, surrounded by extensive and swelling grounds and gardens. The interior is fitted up with galleries, workshops, and music rooms. The sun and the air are allowed to enter at every window, the view of the shrubberies and fields, and groups of labourers, is unobstructed by shatters [sic] or bars; all is clean, quiet attractive. The inmates all seem to be actuated by the common impulse of enjoyment, all are busy, and delighted by being so. The house and all around appears a hive of industry. ...There is in this community no compulsion, no chains, no whips, no corporal punishment, simply because these are proved to be less effectual means of carrying any point than persuasion, emulation, and the desire of obtaining gratification. ... Such is a faithful picture of what may be seen in many institutions, and of what might be seen in all, were asylums conducted as they ought to be.

Politicians may have a determining role in the failure as well as the success of psychiatry. Alfred Hoche, a psychiatrist and neuropathologist, together with Karl Biding, an influential legal scholar, was instrumental in developing the ideology of 'life unworthy of life' but the extermination of so many mentally ill people in Germany would not have occurred without a receptive audience in the general public and the political might of the Nazi party (Friedlander, 1995, chapter 1).

The political abuse of psychiatry has not been limited to Nazi Germany. The Communist abuse of the specialty in Soviet Union is another example (Musto, 2009). Here the intention was not to abuse the mentally ill but to label and 'treat' political dissidents as mentally ill. The abuse of psychiatry or those with mental health problems or learning disability does not need to be political in a narrow sense of the term, as the widespread use of forced sterilization of people with learning disability in countries as diverse as Germany, Sweden, and the United States in the early–middle part of the twentieth century demonstrates (Porter D, 1999, chapter 10).

The destructive effect of politicians or political and other ideologies on psychiatry is not thought by everyone to have occurred only in distant times or places. For example, Jones (1993), a former professor of social policy at York University, England, offers a trenchant critique of what she presents as the destructive effect of libertarian ideology on British psychiatry in the years 1962–1993. The fact that such ideology, which led to a drastic reduction in inpatient bed numbers, was coupled with undoubtedly well-intentioned aims at deinstitutionalization does not soften the blow to those patients and carers who have suffered the consequences (Coid, 1994). Such concerns have not been unique to the United Kingdom. For example, in Denmark a precipitous reduction of number of inpatient psychiatric beds coincided with a doubling of suicide rate between 1970 and 1987 (Shorter, 2007).

Reports from the United States that deinstitutionalization has been succeeded by a state of affairs whereby the largest 'psychiatric hospital' in the country is in the Los Angeles County state prison hospital (Sharfstein, personal communication) suggest that in that country too, perhaps in that country in particular, the libertarian doctrine may have had destructive consequences. Psychiatrists raised early concerns about community care of the severely mentally ill in the United States (Lamb, 2000). It is undoubtedly the case that sometimes when they do sound the alarm, psychiatrists are not heard and this phenomenon in not restricted to the United States (Jones, chapter 4).

Whatever the merits or demerits of past community care policies may have been, they differ crucially from the practices of Nazi Germany and Soviet Communism in being implemented after open debate and in being motivated, in the greater part at the very least, by beneficent ambitions in relation to patients rather than the advancement of a particular authoritarian political system or punitive or evil intent. The interface between political philosophy and psychiatry is interesting and important (Ikkos, Boardman, & Zigmond, 2006) and Jones' fear that neo-liberal economics fuelled much of the libertarian rhetoric (but not all) can not be dismissed out of hand.

Whatever the merits of Jones' critique of libertarianism and its impact on psychiatry, contemporary policymakers continue favouring the provision of mental health services in the community (Knapp, McDaid, Mossialos, & Thornicroft, 2007). The failures of asylum psychiatry, patient preferences, and mental health economics support this. It remains to be established whether the overall judgement of history will differ between the second (asylum) and third (current) community psychiatry. Different times and societies demand different solutions. Paucity of data as well as different conditions makes comparisons difficult (Shorter, 2007). The burden of community psychiatry on carers has not been adequately evaluated. Some authoritative observers are optimistic (Department of Health 2009; European Commission and World Health Organisation 2008). Shorter (2009) singled out the United Kingdom and

Portugal as countries in Europe where most 'spectacular' progress in community psychiatry has been achieved. Recent favourable developments have occurred in times of plenty, and it is at times of paucity of resources that the mentally ill are particularly vulnerable (Birley, 2002; Jones 1994, chapter 7).

The World Psychiatric Association in the Declaration of Madrid in 1996 set forward universal 'ethical standards for the practice of psychiatry' irrespective of local conditions and resources. The most recently updated document includes guidelines on specific situations (World Psychiatric Association, 2005). This, together with a well-established body of knowledge about effective treatments (Tyrer & Silk, 2008) gives hope that the conduct and practice of psychiatrists has much good in common across the globe, even when the pattern of mental health systems in place differs from one country to another.

Professional diversity and psychiatry

Healing the mentally ill has never been the exclusive province of doctors or psychiatrists. Their care has been going on since time immemorial, initially at home and in the temple ('the first community psychiatry'), later in specialist institutions/asylums ('the second community psychiatry') and now, again, increasingly in the community ('the third community psychiatry'). Spirituality, religion, and the clergy have always played a part, and their involvement seems destined to continue (Cook, Powell, & Sims, 2009). Others have also played a part and their contribution is likely to increase in the future.

The York Retreat, founded in 1792, is internationally known as an example of humane early institutional modern mental health care (Jones, 2002, chapter 2). There were no doctors working there at the time. Crucial to its success were George Jepson and Katharine Allen. A married couple, they worked in the employ of the religiously inspired Quaker owners, the Tukes. Jepson and Allen can be described as early forerunners of mental health nurses. The profession of mental health nursing in the United Kingdom has developed with the encouragement of psychiatrists since the 1870s (Bewley, 2008). It is increasingly developing its identity (Department of Health, 2006)

A number of other mental health professions have also developed and have crucial contributions to make, for example, mental health social work, clinical psychology, and occupational therapy. Sometimes their role has been conceived of in opposition to that of the psychiatrist. This has been the case with 'approved social' workers under the Mental Health Act (1983) in England. Sometimes psychologists also give the impression that they may wish to define clinical psychology in opposition to (Bentall, 2004) or to the exclusion of psychiatrists (Kinderman & Tai, 2008). The recent participation of American psychologists (but not psychiatrists) in interrogations of suspected terrorists suggests that no single profession has a monopoly on vice or virtue (Pope & Gutheil, 2009). Maj (2008) has highlighted potential conflicts of interest arising out of researchers' allegiance to a specific school of thought.

Professionalism in psychiatry is enhanced by effective collaboration with others (McQueen, D., St. John-Smith, P., Ikkos, G., et. al, 2009). A recent example of pioneering and effective interprofessional collaboration between mental health professionals at the institutional level (and an important development in the history of psychiatry) is the National Collaborating Centre for Mental Health (NCCMH) (http://www.rcpsych.ac.uk/clinicalservicestandards/nationalcollaboratingcentre.aspx).

Established in 2001, funded by the National Health Service in England and Wales and jointly managed by the British Psychological Society and the Royal College of Psychiatrists, NCCMH issues evidence-based guidance on the management of specific psychiatric disorders or mental health problems under the auspices of the National Institute of Health and Clinical Excellence (NICE) (www.nice.org.uk). The question that NCCMH attempts to answer is not simply whether treatment works but whether treatment gains are such as to justify the National Health Service in England and Wales spending money on it in the context of limited public resources. Although its recommendations may occasionally attract just criticism from practicing psychologists and psychiatrists as well as others, its methodology is consistent with standards advocated by leading thinkers in the field (Sabin & Daniels, 2009). Included are engagement of stakeholders, publicity of procedures, review of values and evidence, health economic as well as clinical effectiveness evaluation, and opportunities to comment and appeal.

The diversity of psychiatry among different countries and the diversity of mental health professionals within the same country have been referred to. The diversity of psychiatrists in different subspecialties also merits attention. It is lamentable that not only the general public but also policymakers and others too often ignore the subspecialties, which are of increasing importance. It is appropriate to refer to them in the context of discussing NCCMH, as this diversity in significant part reflects developments in knowledge/evidence and service delivery.

The European Union of Medical Specialties (UEMS) has separate adult and child and adolescent psychiatry sections (Cox, 2007). A UEMS study concluded that the development of national training accreditation strategies must take precedence over international accreditation in psychiatry (Strachan & Schudel, 2004). This allows considerable freedom to individual countries in the accreditation of subspecialties. The following account relies heavily on Bewley (2008) and the author's personal experience, both centred on the

United Kingdom and particularly the Royal College of Psychiatrists. It is hoped that it will be of general interest both in the similarities and the differences it may suggest in comparisons with other countries. The numbers in parentheses represent the members of the College on 31 July 2009 who identified the particular subspecialty as their primary area of expertise. Although psychiatrists may identify one of the areas below as their primary area of expertise, they may practice across more than one subspecialty. It is important, when reading below, to be aware that in the United Kingdom, psychiatry is a secondary care specialty and much mental health care is actually delivered by general practitioners and other primary care mental health workers, and this has been increasingly the case in recent years and a trend likely to continue.

The largest psychiatric subspecialty is general adult and community psychiatry (6760 members, approximately half the total college number). Forensic psychiatry (1672 members) is probably the earliest other subspecialty. The definition of forensic psychiatry differs from country to country, in some cases referring to specialists who deal with mentally abnormal offenders, whereas in others it extends to all those who specialize in giving evidence to the court, whether in criminal or civil. Esquirol pioneered the use of psychiatric evidence in court in France early in the nineteenth century. The first 'criminal lunatic asylum' in the United Kingdom was established in Dublin, Ireland in 1845 (Appignanessi, 2008, chapter 2). The psychiatry of learning disability is also an early subspecialty, the first 'Asylum for Idiots' having been established in London in 1846 and the first 'Idiot's Act' in 1886 (Faculty of Learning Disability, 882 members).

The first child guidance clinic was established in Boston, USA in the early 1920s. The Child Guidance Section was established in the Royal Medicopsychological Association in 1946 (now the Faculty of Child and Adolescent Psychiatry, 1974 members). Although Alois Alzheimer described the neuropathology of his eponymous dementia in a lecture in 1906 and Felix Post published his seminal paper 'On Some Problems Arising from the Study of Mental Patients ver the Age of 60 Years' in 1945, the Old Age Psychiatry Section was not established within College until 1976 (now the Faculty of Old Age Psychiatry, 2064 members).

In the United Kingdom in addition to the above subspecialties the following are also recognized by the General Medical Council for the purposes of official training accreditation: psychotherapy (719 members), addiction psychiatry (731 members), liaison psychiatry (or psychosomatic medicine, 663 members), rehabilitation psychiatry (535 members), and forensic psychotherapy (54 members).

Psychotherapy is an important element in the practice of all subspecialties of psychiatry. It has a long history beginning as 'moral treatment' in the Retreat and other early asylums, through Freud and psychoanalytic psychotherapy at the beginning of the twentieth century and therapeutic communities after the Second World War to family therapy and cognitive behaviour therapy and other short-term treatments in more recent times. Many psychiatrists, although not identifying this as their primary areas of expertise, have additional specialist postgraduate training in specific types of psychological treatment.

The Royal College of Psychiatrists also recognizes the following as sufficiently distinct areas of knowledge and practice: academic psychiatry (326 members), neuropsychiatry (236 members), perinatal psychiatry, and eating disorders psychiatry. Much, but not all, that is classified as general adult, learning disability, and old age psychiatry might be classified as neuropsychiatry in other countries. Furthermore, some of the work that psychiatrists perform in the United Kingdom might be carried out by different specialists, for example, neurologists and dementia experts.

Conclusion

As Miller (1997) aptly diagnosed, neurology without signs, in other words psychiatry, depends on narrative. However, psychiatry is much more than simply neurology without signs. Narrative, values, culture as well as science (social, psychological, and biological), and clinical skills are crucial to the practice of the specialty. It is a broadly integrative discipline.

Physical illness, mental illness, mental incapacity, mental decline, mental distress, depression, delirium, delusion, hallucination, obsession, addiction, imagined illness, illness denied, medically unexplained symptoms, contrived illness and deceit, self-harm and starvation, offending behaviour, and child abuse are all within the specialty's range. Patients are vulnerable, carers distressed, and the stakes can be very high. Actual experience has not always matched lofty ideals expressed in confident rhetoric.

Ultimately psychiatry depends on society's values and resources, including health care systems. History suggests the psychiatrist must pay increasing attention to understanding values, working in teams and managing systems as well as be proficient in the art and science of direct clinical assessment and treatment. Knowledge has advanced, and more professions are ready to make valuable contributions; complex systems, multidisciplinary, teams and subspecialization have arrived. Society, service users and carers, allied professions, and psychiatrists must all do well to match the standards set by Pinel!

References

Appignanessi, L. (2008). *Mad, Bad and Sad: A History of Women and the Mind Doctors from 1800 to the Present*. London: Virago Press.

Bentall, R. (2004). *Madness Explained: Psychosis and Human Nature*. London: Allen Lane.

Bewley, T. (2008). *Madness to Mental Illness: A History of the Royal College of Psychiatrists*. London: RCPsych Publications.

Bhugra, D. (2008). Renewing psychiatry's contract with society. *Psychiatric Bulletin*, **32**, 281–283.

Birley, J. L. T. (2002). Famine, the distant shadow over French psychiatry. *British Journal of Psychiatry*, **180**, 298–299.

BMA Health Policy and Economic Research Unit. (2008). *The Role of the Doctor – Building on the Past, Looking to the Future*. London: British Medical Association.

Care Services Improvement Partnership, Royal College of Psychiatrists, Social Care Institute. (2007). A Common Purpose: Recovery in Future Mental Health Services. Retrieved 19 June 2010 from http://www.scie.org.uk.

Coid, J. W. (1994). Editorial: The Christopher Clunis enquiry. *Psychiatric Bulletin*, **18**, 449–452.

Cook, C., Powell, A., & Sims, A. (2009). *Spirituality and Psychiatry*. London: RCPsych Publications.

Cox, J. (2007). European psychiatry: Moving towards integration and harmony. *World Psychiatry*, **6**, 54–56.

Craddock, N., Antebi, D., & Attenburrow, M. J., et al. (2008). Wake-up call for British psychiatry. *British Journal of Psychiatry*, **193**, 6–9.

Department of Health. (2009a). *From Values to Action: The Chief Medical Officer's Review of Mental Health Nursing*. London: Department of Health Publications.

Department of Health. (2009b). *New Horizons: Towards a Shared Vision for Mental Health-Consultation*. London: Department of Health Publications.

European Commission and World Health Organisation. (2008). *Policies and Practices for Mental Health in Europe*. World Health Organization.

Friedlander, H. (1995). *The Origins of Nazi Genocide from Euthanasia to the Final Solution*. Chapel Hill and London: University of North Carolina Press.

Fulford, K. W. M., Thornton, T., & Graham, G. (2006). *Values, Ethics and Mental Health Practice* (Part IV in Oxford Textbook of Philosophy and Psychiatry). Oxford: Oxford University Press.

Gelder, M. G., Andreasen, N. C., Lopez-Ibor Jr, J. J., & Geddes, J. R. (2009). *New Oxford Textbook of Psychiatry* (2nd ed.). Oxford: Oxford University Press.

Higgins, E. S., & George, M. S. (2007). *The Neuroscience of Clinical Psychiatry: The Pathophysiology of Behaviour and Mental Illness*. New York: Wolters Kluwer and Lippincott Williams and Wilkins.

Ikkos, G. (2003). Engaging patients/users as teachers of interview skills to new doctors in psychiatry. *Psychiatric Bulletin*, **27**, 312–315.

Ikkos, G. (2005). Mental health services users involvement: Teaching doctors successfully. *Primary Care Mental Health*, **3**, 139–144.

Ikkos, G., Boardman, J., & Zigmond, A. (2006). Talking liberties: John Rawls' theory of justice and psychiatric practice. *Advances in Psychiatric Treatment*, **12**, 202–213.

International Labour Organization. (2008). Retrieved 19 June 2010 from www.ilo.org/public/english/bureau/stat/isco/draftdoc.htm.

Jones, K. (2002). *Asylums and After: A Revised History of Mental Health Services*. London: Jessica Kingsley.

Kinderman, P., & Tai. S. (Eds) (2008). *Psychological Health and Wellbeing: A New Ethos and a New Service Structure for Mental Health: A Report of the Working Group on Psychological Health and Wellbeing*. Leicester: British Psychological Society.

Knapp, M., McDaid, D., Mossialos, E., & Thornicroft, G. (2007). Mental health policy and practice across Europe: An overview. In M. Knapp, D. McDaid, E. Mossialos, & G. Thornicroft (Eds), *Mental Health Policy and Practice across Europe: The Future Direction of Mental Health Care* (pp. 1–14). Maidenhead: McGraw Hill Open University Press.

Kuczewski, M. (2006). The problem with evaluating professionalism. In D. Wear, & J. M. Aultman (Eds), *Professionalism in Medicine: Critical Perspectives* (pp.185–198). New York: Springer.

Lamb, H. R. (2000). The 1978 conference on the chronic mental patient. *Psychiatric Services*, **51**, 874–878.

Maj, M. (2008). Non-financial conflicts of interest in psychiatric research, *British Journal of Psychiatry*, **193**, 91–92.

Magliano, L., McDaid, D., Kirkwood, S., & Berzins, K. (2007). Carers and families of people with mental health problems. In M. Knapp, D. McDaid, E. Mossialos, & G. Thornicroft (Eds), *Mental Health Policy and Practice across Europe: The Future Direction of Mental Health Care* (pp. 374–396). Maidenhead: McGraw Hill Open University Press.

Marneros, A., (2008). Psychiatry's 200th birthday. *British Journal of Psychiatry*, **193**, 1–3.

McQueen, D., Ikkos, G., St John Smith, P., Kemp, M., Munk-Jorgensen, P., Michael, A., (2010). Psychiatry's Contract with Society: what do clinical psychiatrists expect? Ch 8. in Bhugra, D., Malik, A. Ikkos, G. (Eds), 2010 *Psychiatry's Contract with Society* Oxford University Press.

McQueen, D., St John Smith, P., Ikkos, G., Kemp, M., Munk-Jorgensen, P., Michael A., (2009). Psychiatric Professionalism, Multidisciplinary Teams and Clinical Practice, *European Psychiatric Review*, **2**(2) 50–56.

Medical Professionalism Project. (2002). Medical professionalism in the new millennium: A physicians' charter. *The Lancet*, **359**, 520–522.

Musto, D. F. (2009). A historical perspective. In S. Bloch, S. A. Green (Eds), *Psychiatric Ethics* (pp.). Oxford: Oxford University Press.

Pope, K., & Gutheil, T. (2009). The interrogation of detainees: How the ethics of psychologists and doctors differ. *British Medical Journal*, **338**, 1178–1179.

Pormann, P. E., & Savage-Smith, E. (2007). *Medieval Islamic Medicine*. Edinburgh: Edinburgh University Press.

Porter, D. (1999). *Health, Civilisation and the State: A History of Public Health from Ancient to Modern Times*. London: Routledge.

Porter, R. (1997). *The Greatest Benefit to Mankind: A Medical History of Humanity from Antiquity to the Present*. London: Fontana Press.

Porter, R. (2002). *Madness: A Brief History*. Oxford: Oxford University Press.

Post, F. (1945). On some problems arising from a study of mental patients over the age of 60 years. *Journal of Mental Science*, **90**, 554–565.

Rivett, T. (2006). *From Cradle to Grave: Fifty years of the NHS*. London: King's Fund.

Rose, D., & Lucas, J. (2007). The user and survivor movement in Europe. In M. Knapp, D. McDaid, E. Mossialos, & G. Thornicroft (Eds), *Mental Health Policy and Practice across Europe: The Future Direction of Mental Health Care* (pp. 336–355). Maidenhead: McGraw Hill Open University Press.

Royal College of Physicians. (2005). Doctors in society: Medical professionalism in a changing world. London: Royal College of Physicians.

Royal College of Psychiatrists. (2009). *Good Psychiatric Practice* (3rd ed). London: RCPsych Publications.

Royal College of Psychiatrists Social Inclusion Scoping Group. (2009). *Mental Health and Social Inclusion; Making Mental Health Services Fit for the 21st Century, Position Statement*. London: RCPsych Publications.

Sabin, J. E., & Daniels, N. (2009). Allocation of mental health resources. In S. Bloch, & S. A. Green (Eds), *Psychiatric Ethics* (pp. 111–126). Oxford: Oxford University Press.

Sibbald, B., & Knight R. (2008). Should primary care be nurse led? *British Medical Journal*, **337**, 658–659.

Shorter, E. (2007). The historical development of mental health services in Europe. In M. Knapp, D. McDaid, E. Mossialos, & G. Thornicroft (Eds), *Mental Health Policy and Practice Across Europe: The Future Direction of Mental Health Care* (pp. 15–33). Maidenhead: McGraw Hill Open University Press.

St John-Smith, P., McQueen, D., Ikkos, G., Kemp, M., Munk-Jorgensen, P., & Michael, A. (2009). Psychiatric professionalism, multidisciplinary teams and clinical practice. *European Psychiatric Review*, **2**, 50–54.

St John-Smith, P., McQueen, D., Michael, A., et al. (2009). The trouble with NHS psychiatry in England. *Psychiatric Bulletin*, **33**, 219–225.

Strachan, J. G., & Schudel, W. J. (2004). Accreditation of European training schemes in psychiatry. *Psychiatric Bulletin*, **28**, 19–20.

Tyrer, P., & Silk, K. R. Eds (2008). *Effective Treatment in Psychiatry*. Cambridge: Cambridge University Press.

Williams, R., & Kerfoot, M (2005). Setting the scene: perspectives on the history of and policy of adolescent mental health services in the UK. In R. Williams, & M. Kerfoot (Eds), *Child and Adolescent Mental Health Services; Strategy, Planning, Delivery and Evaluation* (pp. 1–38). Oxford: Oxford University Press.

World Psychiatric Association. Madrid Declaration on Ethical Standards for Psychiatric Practice (2005). Retrieved 19 June 2010 from http://www.wpanet.org/content/madrid-ethic-engish.shtml

Yousif, M., (2009). Carers and Medical Training, Health Services Journal, e-version, 26 October.

Chapter 3

Professions, related occupations, and ethics

Robin Downie

There has been a great deal of writing during the past two decades on the professions and professional values, the basic reason being that those who see themselves as belonging to a profession also see themselves as under threat. This threat comes from various sources. First, the general public is no longer willing to tolerate poor service, and various bodies have been set up to monitor the activities of given professions. Second, this public disquiet has been picked up by governments of all political persuasions, who have seized the opportunity to remove or restrict the independent nature of the professions. 'Seized the opportunity' is an appropriate expression because the professions have traditionally enjoyed a measure of public esteem not usually accorded to politicians, who have consequently welcomed the opportunity to harness professional activities 'in the public interest'. Third, journalists and TV interviewers (who themselves have a low public standing) make the most of any professional scandals, especially if they involve the medical profession. Fourth, despite the slow lowering of the status of the professions, many occupations not traditionally regarded as 'professions' wish to place themselves in that category. It is therefore not surprising that the traditional professions are on the defensive. To investigate the matter we must consider the criteria in terms of which an occupation can be seen as a profession, how many occupations satisfy the criteria, and whether the occupational category of 'profession' is worth preserving.

Definitions and evaluative criteria

The first difficulty concerns the sort of definition that would be helpful. There is a large sociological literature on the professions, but sociologists tend to identify professions in terms of descriptive or factual criteria such as at least five years of training, a code of ethics, an annual conference, remuneration by fees or salary rather than wages, and so on. Now it might be possible to define a profession using such criteria, but they do not really advance our understanding of why a profession might have a valuable contribution to make to the community, or why professional decisions typically involve judgements of value. I shall therefore suggest evaluative criteria as a basis for a definition. However, as we shall see, these criteria have implications that are contentious if they are regarded as constituting the necessary and sufficient conditions of a definition.

The first of the evaluative criteria is that a profession must be a learned occupation; it has a basis of knowledge and skills. This is perhaps the criterion which, historically, would originally have distinguished a profession from other occupations; the schoolmaster, the clergyman, and the doctor were the main scholars of an earlier epoch. However, now many occupations have a basis in knowledge and skills, and this criterion can therefore be no more than necessary to distinguish a profession; it certainly is not sufficient.

Not only must a professional have knowledge and skills, he or she must know when, how, and how much to exercise the skills. For example, the skilled surgeon may be able to carry out the complex operation, but he or she must decide whether the operation ought to be attempted. This kind of decision is of a different order; it involves judgements of moral value. What is the balance of risks and harms? Has the patient consented to the risks? What are the long-term prospects of recovery? And so on. This complex mixture of the technical and the ethical ideally requires that the surgeon be broadly educated as well as technically skilled. We can therefore make education in humane values a second criterion for a profession.

This second criterion requires some expansion. What are the differences between being trained to have skills and being educated in humane values? This, of course, is a major topic on its own, but a few points can helpfully be made. First, the person educated in humane values has a broad cognitive perspective and is able to see the significance of social work, teaching, medicine, or the law, for example, in a total way of life. Second, the person of humane education has a continual curiosity about the world, a desire to develop the skills throughout a working life, and connectedly is aware of the standards of work, which must be satisfied. Here we have the familiar idea of a 'professional job', or a 'job well done'. Third, the idea of a humane education embodies the idea of ethics. It is possible to be trained to pick pockets, as in Dickens' *Oliver Twist*, but a humane education is necessarily directed to worthwhile ends. Here we have the idea of standards of behaviour, of 'being professional' in one's approach to a client, patient, or student. Fourth, the broadly educated person has a flexibility of mind that enables her/him to see things in a variety of ways. The philosopher of education, R.S. Peters (1967), puts the point in a memorable way: 'To be educated is not to have arrived; it is to travel with a different view'.

A good analogy that brings out the nature of the fourth attribute of the educated person is given by the twentieth century philosopher Wittgenstein (1953). His example is of a fly in a glass bottle. The fly buzzes against the glass and cannot escape, but there is no stopper in the bottle. If the fly changed direction, it could fly straight out. The person of flexible mind is the one who can show the fly the way out of the bottle! The point here is that there tends to be a grey uniformity about professional education: nowadays it is forced into the mould of aims and objectives, powerpoint presentations, and bullet points. No doubt there are merits in this, but the price is stereotyping and a suppression of individuality. To a layman like myself it is not unamusing that psychiatrists (and doctors more generally), who rightly stress the importance of communication and listening skills, are themselves unable to deliver or follow a talk without the use of 'powerpoint'. The main messages must be arranged in bullet points or spooned into boxes! This may make for easy assimilation but not for complexity of thought. In contrast, the educated professional must have the ability to think differently. As J.S. Mill (1969, p. 188) puts it in his essay *On Liberty*: '[human nature] is not a machine built after a model... but a tree, which requires to grow and develop on all sides, according to the tendency of the inward forces which make it a living thing.' Professional education must avoid the idea that one size fits all. If the first requirement for a profession is a base of knowledge and skills, the second is that the knowledge and skills must be developed in a long-term programme that includes broad and ethical perspectives on the profession and its skills and does not stifle individuality.

All professions offer a public service to clients, patients, students, or the like. In more detail this service is offered through a special relationship. This is the third factor in my attempted definition. What is meant here by a relationship? The word 'relationship' can be used in two ways. It can refer to the bonds that hold two people together, or it can refer to their attitudes to each other. For example, if we see two people together, we might ask what is the relationship between them, and receive answers such as father and son, colleagues, husband and wife, teacher and pupil, doctor and patient, and so on. To characterize a relationship in this way is to ask about what I am calling the 'bonds'. But, we might also ask what kind of relationship do Bloggs and his son have, and be told, 'Bloggs has great affection for his son, but his son has nothing but contempt for his father.' Or we might say of a husband and wife that their relationship is deteriorating, or of that between a doctor and a patient that the patient trusts the doctor and the doctor respects the patient. Answers of that kind characterize a relationship in terms of attitudes. A professional relationship requires attitude as well as bond.

The bonds in a professional relationship are decided by the governing body, for example, by the GMC. It is necessary that there should be special bonds between the professional and the client because of the inequality in the relationship. In brief, the client, student, or patient is vulnerable and needs the protection of the bond. In general, we might say that the bond takes the form of a role-relationship in which the professional and the client have rights and duties laid down by the governing body. For example, a doctor, lawyer, or accountant might need to know various intimate details about the client to be able to offer the service. The client must be reassured that no untoward use will be made of this information. Hence, duties of confidentiality are imposed on the professional. Again, a teacher or a tutor will need to criticize the work of a pupil or student. However, the fact that they are in a role-relationship with respect to each other creates insulation against the wrong sort of emotional side-effects of criticism. Doctors are told that 'the patient is a person,' and so on. Yes, but they are persons in a role-relationship when they are dealing with a professional. Furthermore, the nature of the role is laid down by the professional body and obviously reflects the values of the profession. In other words, ethics enters a profession through the professional bond.

Ethics also enters through the professional attitude. We can say that the attitude must reflect awareness of the vulnerability of the client, patient, or student. Often the professional attitude is described by a term such as 'beneficence.' In *Canterbury Tales,* Chaucer (1957, p. 425) characterizes the poor Parson as follows:

> Benigne he was, and wonder diligent,
> and in adversitee full pacient

The pathology of beneficence is paternalism, a word from which contemporary professionals shy away. Of course, in a sense the doctor does know best about your medical interests. Why otherwise do you consult the doctor? Nowadays, information and the patient's right to give or withhold consent in the light of that information makes the term 'paternalism' less appropriate. There are other sorts of problems in other professions; however, whatever the details in the composition of the attitudes involved in the professional relationship, they clearly involve moral values.

A fourth feature of the professions is that professional leaders have a moral duty to speak out on matters of public policy as it affects their profession. For example, judges have a duty to speak out on matters of sentencing, psychiatrists on matters of mental health policy, teachers' leaders and vice-chancellors on education, and architects on housing policies, planning permission, conservation, and the like. Governments do not always like this. There has been a tendency for governments of both the right and the left to resist the influence of the professions, seeing that influence as a kind of threat to their political positions. Campaigns against the professions are easy to mount with support from the media, for there have been high-profile scandals that encourage public opinion to turn against the professions and depict them as 'elitist', monopolistic, and unaccountable. However, 'being accountable' generally means being subject to a government agenda, to meet targets, or the like. It is good for a society if there is a measure of political pluralism, and the professions can be one source of basic political values.

If the professions are to be a reliable source of independent advice, they must be self-regulating. This is the fifth criterion that an occupation must satisfy to be a profession. Here I part company with the Royal College of Physicians of London (RCP). In 2005 the College published the report of a working party entitled *Doctors in Society: Medical Professionalism in a Changing Society*. The RCP recognizes that 'self-regulation' had once been a criterion for an occupation to be a profession and that 'many doctors would defend it as a sensible and practical way to govern the profession' (Royal College of Physicians, 2005, p. 516), but they propose to abandon it. Why? One argument might be that it is increasingly difficult for any profession to satisfy this criterion. Most professions are dependent on government finance or large pharmaceutical companies. But that is not the argument used by the RCP. What they say is: '[Self-regulation] is irrelevant to the essential values and behaviours that underpin professional practice' (p. 516). However, as it seems to me, self-regulation is of the essence for professional values. The reason is the obvious one that if you pay the piper, you want to call the tune, and this is precisely what governments have increasingly been doing to the professions. They impose targets, curricula, and policies, all with a political agenda in mind. Despite the high esteem in which medicine is held by the general public this has not effectively been resisted. Whereas it is a good thing if there are lay members of a governing body it is a bad thing if self-regulation breaks down entirely. To resist external bullying, courage is needed – an underestimated moral value of great relevance to the professions and not included in the RCP list of values.

Of course, it is often argued against the self-regulation of professions that they must be 'accountable'. Yes, but accountable to whom? Professions typically have governing bodies concerned with discipline and ethics. These governing bodies have lay members, and lay members can bring an independence from the professional ethos. Of course, there is a danger that lay members will tend to go along with the views of the professional representatives. However, the alternative to self-regulation is government interference through appointed managers. The general public and the media respond favourably to political assertions to the effect that the professions must be 'accountable'. But it is not so widely realized that this largely amounts to a managerial/government takeover, with its attendant targets and highly paid bureaucracy. Therefore, it is to be hoped that the professions will have the courage to hold on to the remnants of self-regulation and to the right to comment on government policies. The judiciary has to a great extent stood up to governments but doctors have to a great extent caved in, as can be seen in the RCP Report.

Family resemblances

So far I have suggested five criteria that an occupation must satisfy if it is to count as a profession: knowledge and skills; a broad framework of values stemming from a humane education; a public service provided through a special relationship; a duty to comment on matters of public policy; and professional self-regulation. Now these criteria seem plausible enough, but if we regard them as constituting a definition – a set of necessary and sufficient conditions for an occupation to count as a profession – we are faced with some implications that are likely to be unpalatable to many who consider that they are in professions. I have now reached the point in the argument that might be considered contentious. For if we regard the criteria as constituting a definition, we have ruled out as professions at least the following occupations: civil servants, the armed forces, journalists, the police, scientists, writers, musicians, actors, airline pilots, estate agents, politicians, and so on. There may be at least two reasons to rule them out as professions, despite the fact that they offer a valuable public service. The first is that they do not offer their service through a special relationship; second is that at least some may not satisfy the first two criteria: they may lack a sufficient knowledge base, and they may lack the broad educational framework.

There are two possible approaches to this implication of the criteria. The first is to accept the implication and say that some occupations offer a public service, and professions are a subset of these; they are public service occupations that have a more developed knowledge base and offer the service through a special relationship. The other approach, perhaps preferable, is to drop the idea of a strict definition, of being 'absolutely clear' about what we are going to mean by the term 'profession', and say instead that we are dealing with a range of occupations that have a 'family resemblance' (Wittgenstein, 1953). Members of a large family do not all have the same features, but they have a number of features which, as it were, overlap and enable us to recognize someone as belonging to that family. This approach follows from the point that occupations develop over the years: some become professions, and others may cease to be such if the public no longer needs the service. For example, surgeons or dentists are now clearly in professions but it was not always so.

Professions and business

Nevertheless, although I have made the concept of a profession more fluid the question remains whether every sort of occupation can be included. One important contrast is often made between the professions, widely or narrowly construed, and business. How valid is that comparison, and how can the values of each be compared and contrasted?

There is certainly an overlap, family resemblances, between some of the criteria for a business and those I have proposed for a profession. For example, business leaders would nowadays stress the importance of skills and a broad education. Business and industry employ not only those with technical and scientific qualifications but also graduates in the arts. A broad educated vision is regarded as necessary for successful business. Again, business leaders perform a valuable social function by speaking out on matters of employment, damaging taxation, environmental issues, and the like. The voices of bodies such as the Confederation of British Industry are respected by governments and the population more generally. Large businesses also fulfil an important social function by sponsoring the arts and sport.

Nevertheless, it is a common view that the crucial difference between the professions, broadly or narrowly conceived, and business is this: the professions are beneficently directed towards clients, patients, or students, whereas business is self-interestedly directed towards customers. The classic statement of the self-interested nature of business is provided by Adam Smith, Professor of Moral Philosophy at Glasgow University (1752–63). In his great work *The Wealth of Nations,* he writes as follows (1976, p. 118):

> In almost every other race of animals, each individual, when it is grown up to maturity, is entirely independent, and in the natural state has occasion for the assistance of no other living creature. But man has almost constant occasion for the help of his brethren, and it is in vain for him to expect it from their benevolence only. He is more likely to prevail if he can interest their self-love in his favour, and show them that it is their own advantage to do for him what he requires of them. It is not from the benevolence of the butcher, the brewer, or the baker that we expect our dinner, but from their regard to their own self-interest. We address ourselves, not to their humanity, but to their self-love, and never talk to them of our own necessities, but of their advantages.

This alleged contrast, between the beneficence of the professions and the self-interest of those in business, can have unfortunate effects. It can create a sense of moral superiority in the professions. For example, the RCP Report on medical professionalism makes the extraordinary claim that 'altruism' is a value of the profession. It is true that they indicate that this was controversial, even within the working party, but they wish to retain the value on the grounds that many physicians, trainees, and the Department of Health agreed with the statement: 'Medical practice requires altruism.' Indeed, 75% of the Fellows and members of the RCP agreed with the statement. Therefore, it must be obviously true! It seems strange that a profession committed to evidence should draw its evidence on how their practice should be evaluated solely from their evaluation of themselves. If doctors are to be considered altruistic simply for doing their job, for which they receive a very large remuneration, what is the appropriate term for lifeboat men who (in addition to their daily job) put their lives on the line for others, for no remuneration? No one doubts that doctors are hardworking, but so also are teachers (consider inner-city schools), policemen, and orchestral musicians. However, they do not make embarrassingly extravagant moral claims about their conduct. If doctors wish to retain their high position in public esteem they should drop their persistent claims to the moral high ground. Chaucer's description of the Doctour of Phisik should not be forgotten (1957, p. 424):

> *For gold in phisik is a cordial,*
> *Therfore he lovede gold in special.*

Bernard Shaw's views (1926, Act 1) should also be noted as an antidote to self-congratulation: 'All professions are conspiracies against the laity.'

In reply to the self-congratulation of the professions there are often aggressive responses from business, such as 'We live in the real world and not in an ivory tower,' or 'We earn the wealth of the country on which the professions depend.' How valid is the contrast between the professions and business implicit in Adam Smith's claim? To answer the question we must distinguish the point at which a service is provided or an item sold in the market, and the point at which prices and fees or salary levels are fixed. It is certainly the case that professionals attempt to provide a service to fit the needs or wants of their clients or patients. However, the same is also true of those in business. For example, if I am buying a new computer, I will typically receive good advice for the model that best suits my needs and price range. Certainly, there are unscrupulous salespersons persuading me to buy what is not in my interests, but equally there are unscrupulous professionals who may try to persuade me into frivolous litigation or unnecessary, sometimes even harmful, medical treatment. (Consider some cosmetic surgery.) Now the fact that I expect and most often receive good advice and choice in a free market at the point of service delivery is quite compatible with saying that at the point at which prices are fixed, a business person will consider what the market will stand by way of prices. No altruism here! But, equally, professional bodies fix fees or salaries at a level they think the market or a government will tolerate. Otherwise they bargain with governments to maximize the interests of their members. No altruism here either! Hence, Adam Smith's contrast between the self-interest of a free market and the benevolence of the professions is too simplistic.

There is, however, one important difference between a transaction in the free market and a professional encounter. Suppose that I wish to buy a pair of stout shoes for walking along country lanes. I try various pairs and then my eye lights on a pair of shiny patent leather shoes and I decide to buy them. The salesperson will certainly tell me that the shiny shoes will get scratched quickly and wear out in rough lanes and are not at all suitable for my stated purposes. However, if I persist and put the money down, the shoe sales person has no duty to refuse the sale. Having given honest information and advice, the salesperson hands the responsibility for the purchase to the customer. That is part of the market mechanism. The question is: can that mechanism be carried over into a professional encounter? It cannot, unless the whole idea of a profession is abandoned (Downie & Randall, 2008). The professional integrity and responsibility of the doctor, teacher, architect, and so on entail that their judgement about what is the appropriate service must remain paramount. As professionals they are committed to offer only those services that are in the best interests of their clients or patients. Of course, the client can refuse the service – that is the client's responsibility – but if professionals submit to a client's demands against their professional judgement, then they have committed a cardinal sin against the profession. There is therefore at least one important difference between a professional relationship and one in a free market.

It follows from the above difference that there can be problems of an ethical kind for professionals employed in industry or business. These problems are common to the extent that many professionals are in fact employees of large business concerns. For example, engineers will have certain professional standards concerned with the safety and efficiency of products. However, the achievement of a high professional standard may well conflict with the aim of the business to make a profit for shareholders. In medicine the problem can be that of the medical director who has to meet the targets imposed by chief executives and indirectly by governments. At this point it is easy to say that professionals should never compromise their professional standards. But whistle-blowers never tend to do well in their subsequent career, and many will have families. For example, chief executives of hospital trusts have a large say in applications for merit awards and can easily provide lukewarm support for consultants who have opposed their policies. This is an area where some sort of mechanism should be established by government to safeguard the interests of professionals and the general public.

A second sort of conflict that can arise is in the area of the ownership of knowledge. The tendency, perhaps the duty, of a professional is to publish information and new ideas for the general good but businesses may wish to retain these advances as trade secrets. Despite the overlaps, or the family resemblances between the professions and business, there are therefore clearly significant sources of moral tension, and there is no general way of solving these; moral decisions will be specific to the specific situations.

Professions, trades, crafts, and caring about what you are doing

I have suggested that there are family resemblances between the professions narrowly conceived and broadly conceived, and that, despite crucial differences, there are also resemblances between the professions and business. I wish in conclusion to suggest that these resemblances extend also to those engaged in crafts and other occupations not usually considered professions. The idea of a 'job well done', of high standards of work and behaviour being satisfied, can extend to trades as well as to traditional professions. The idea that the traditional professions have a monopoly of ethics is simply self-deception; after all, Jesus was a carpenter. An excellent description of the professional attitude, and its accompanying ethics, is provided by an account of motorcycle maintenance. In his novel, Robert Pirsig (1974, pp. 26–27) describes the attitudes implicit in technical manuals and in his experience of some mechanics as a 'spectator' attitude:

> These were spectator manuals. It was built into the format of them. Implicit in every line is the idea that 'here is the machine, isolated in time and in space from everything else in the universe. It has no relationship to you, you have no relationship to it. …' And it occurred to me that there is no manual that deals with the real business of motorcycle maintenance, the most important aspect of all. Caring about what you are doing is considered either unimportant or taken for granted.

Professions take note! It may be more important for psychiatrists in their own contexts to unpack the phrase – 'caring about what you are doing' – than to defend the extensive and vulnerable frontier of 'professionalism'.

References

Chaucer, G. (1389/1957). *The Canterbury Tales, Prologue*. Oxford: Oxford University Press.
Downie, R. S., & Randall, F. (2008). Choice and responsibility. *Clinical Medicine*, **8**, 182–185.
Mill, J. S. (1859/1969). *On Liberty*. London: Collins.
Peters, R. S. (Ed.) (1967). *The Concept of Education*. Oxford: Oxford University Press.
Pirsig, R. (1974). *Zen and the Art of Motorcycle Maintenance*. New York: The Bodley Head.

Royal College of Physicians: Report of a Working Party. (2005). Doctors in society: Medical professionalism in a changing world. *Clinical Medicine*, **5**, 516.

Shaw, B. (1906/1925). *The Doctor's Dilemma* (Act 1). London: Constable.

Smith, A. (1776/1976). *The Wealth of Nations*. Hammondsworth: Pelican Classics.

Wittgenstein, L. (1953*). Philosophical Investigations*. Oxford: Blackwell.

Chapter 4

What is expected of doctors?

Lord Victor Adebowale

Introduction

A wider point about the world of psychiatry and psychiatrists is that psychiatry is a club to which most of the population does not belong. Although people may be becoming more psychologically aware, they are not becoming more psychiatrically aware. The popular usage of terms such as closure, denial, and over-compensation demonstrates that people are more and more interested in understanding their own minds. Psychology is rapidly becoming the most popular A level subject and a new glossy magazine called *Psychologies* epitomizes the trend. Yet this does not seem to have translated across to psychiatry. Census data over many years show a high level of consultant vacancies, around 11%, although the figure has gone down since. Only 4% to 5% of graduate doctors choose psychiatry, not nearly enough to meet demand (RCP, 2006). 'In the Psychiatrist's Chair' on BBC Radio 4 has been the only popular reference point in the United Kingdom, which unashamedly uses the term psychiatry or psychiatrist. The only television programme that does present psychiatrists takes much of its humour from their own neuroses: Frasier and Niles Crane are consistently depicted as pompous, elitist professionals, out of touch with real life concerns.

Stigma: Underlying a lot of coverage of psychiatry, psychiatric problems and psychiatric patients is stigma. People seem to be uncomfortable with psychiatry and its practitioners, and this discomfit manifests itself in the public domain. Psychiatrists, as scientists, and as professionals, already operate in a sphere that few understand and something which most find remote, abstruse, and intimidating. However, although professionals and scientists to some extent have always been viewed as elitist and conspiratorial, the problem in many ways is a considerably more knotty one for psychiatrists. The reasons for this are several, and they centre around one maxim that is pleasantly simple to express: that mental illness is scary. The fact that mental illness is scary means that psychiatrists have to work harder than other professionals to counteract the perception of them as remote and inaccessible. For one-third of the public, it is important that scientists listen to or share their concerns (IPSOS-MORI, 2005). Paul Sieghart(1985)demonstrated that people want professionals to behave altruistically when there are ethical dilemmas: to put the patient's interest first. These expectations which are incumbent on all professionals are increasingly weighty when we talk about mental health. Yet patients and their families still report that basic communication from psychiatrists is lacking.

Therefore, psychiatrists work in an area that is intellectually difficult and complex and of which few members of the public have any understanding; and coupled with this is a failure to articulate this sphere adequately to patients, their carers, or to the wider public. This lack of transparency contributes to the perception of prejudice, and generates fear.

These are factors which I consider to have contributed to the distrust of psychiatry and psychiatrists and their marginalization in favour of more popular approaches to mental well-being, such as psychology. In the next section, the nature of the challenge to the profession will be discussed; in the third section some of the good practice which is already happening in psychiatry will be highlighted. However, it is worth noting that it not only needs to be more widespread but that it must become the norm for mental health professionals. It must also, of course, be perceived as the norm by the general public. In the last section, I argue that psychiatrists are best placed to deliver on these issues in the mental health system because of their unique skill set, and in fact that if they do not they will be risking not only the credibility of their profession but also the mental health of the nation.

Why do people distrust the mental health system?

First, psychiatry has from its inception been hugely vulnerable to misuse for political purposes, which gives us historical reasons to distrust it. The Royal College of Psychiatrists itself has spearheaded the exposure of the abuse of psychiatry in the Soviet Union, and many of its leading members have been exerting pressure on various international organizations about similar concerns in China and elsewhere. Having said this, in Russia, 'punitive psychiatry' is still reportedly practised against political dissidents (*Daily Telegraph*, 14 August 2007). Not so long ago in this country, Victorian asylums were used arbitrarily to lock up the mentally well, as the recently highlighted case of Jean Gambell illustrates: sectioned under the 1890 Lunacy Act for stealing two shillings in 1937 – found only in September 2008 by her remaining family. Foucault's Great Confinement was not restricted to the seventeenth century. In *Madness and Civilization*, Foucault identfied enormous houses of confinement that designated 'the same homeland to the poor, to the unemployed, to prisoners, and to the insane' (Foucault, 2001). The act of pathologizing (and imprisoning) difference from the social 'norm' is rooted in psychiatry's history. Psychiatry is, historically, easy to distrust, and the onus is on psychiatrists to rebalance the scales that tilt against it. It has often failed in the past with those two central tenets of professionalism to which are referred above: listening to and sharing the patient's concerns. Psychiatry must prove it is trustworthy and needs to earn this. This is not a given.

Second, as well as people being scared of the mental health system, they are scared of the mentally ill. Only 19% of people agreed that they would be happy living next door to a person with a mental health problem (YouGov, 2007). There is a highly emotive response when a person with a psychiatric diagnosis commits murder or manslaughter. Quiet voices identifying the inherent challenges in managing highly complex illnesses are not usually heard in the crowd, and mental health professionals, including psychiatrists, are the first to be blamed. Doctors are not so immediately blamed when managing complex physical illnesses.

Third, there are comparatively increased levels of scepticism in certain sections of the community. It is essential for these groups to be better engaged with the mental health system for it to fulfil its obligations to patients. It is a sad fact, for example, that may of the black and minority ethnic (BME) populations in the United Kingdom perceive the mental health system to be systematically racist. There is enough evidence to support their views in reports such as 'Breaking the Circles of Fear' (Sainsbury Trust), 'Inside Outside' (Department of Health) and the Inquiry into the death of David Bennett . There is also academic evidence: Bhui et al., report (2003)in a review that calculated a pooled odds ratio of 4.31 for Black inpatients in comparison with White inpatients compulsorily admitted. There was a strong evidence base for a relative excess of compulsory admissions of Black people, even after adjusting for potential confounders such as age, gender, socio-economic status, past admissions, and police involvement. The Count Me In census presents a consistently bleak picture year in, year out. The 2007 census confirmed that Black and White/Black Mixed groups were more likely to be detained under the Mental Health Act compared with the average for all inpatients by up to 38% (Commission for Healthcare Audit and Inspection, 2007).

The population of the United Kingdom is becoming and will continue to become more ethnically complex. More of the patients will be from BME communities. Quite aside from the moral and social arguments for change, there is a huge financial cost – and a natural limit – to increased detention rates, as we have seen from the ever increasing prison population. These examples of BME communities provide a useful illustration of the increased scepticism. Despite the extremely high prevalence of mental health problems among people in prison, there is little access to psychological therapies; older people and children are also less likely to be offered talking therapies (Mental Health Foundation, 2006). These continuing inequalities will continue to precipitate negative attitudes towards mental health services. However, it is well known where there are gaps in the mental health system, as are the demographics of people who are falling through them. Yet the perception of inaction from mental health professionals, including psychiatrists, remains. Such inaction is bound to add to the distrust and stigma.

What is the challenge to psychiatry?

> To say that a man is made up of certain chemical elements is a satisfactory description only for those who intend to use him as a fertilizer.

Hermann Joseph Muller (1890–1967), US geneticist, winner of 1946 Nobel Prize for Medicine

The three reasons identified here that have eroded trust in the profession are by no means exhaustive, but they do serve to indicate the scale of the challenge to psychiatry's image, to its diagnostic framework and to its cost. It is important to note that there are two potential challenges to psychiatry: the first is about how psychiatry actually works (practice problem) and the second is how the public (and demographic sections as noted above within it) thinks it works (perception problem). Psychiatrists must be open about both these problems – explain them and express their views clearly.

The key to the practice problem lies in the fact that, as Bhui and Bhugra (2002) have pointed out, uniformity of medical training across cultures is assumed to lead to uniformity in skills and values. Yet this is much less clear in mental health than in illnesses that have demonstrable physical pathologies and abnormalities. There is greater variation in explanatory models in mental health and the health professional's own explanatory model of illness and its influence on his or her practice has not received adequate attention (Bhui & Bhugra, 2002).

On the one hand, psychiatry is seen as too focused on the medical model of disease and cure (usually with medication) rather than on the disability model, which views patients as individuals living with problems that they need help and care to manage. Medication then becomes one of a number of things that people living with mental health challenges need. On the other hand, psychological and social causative factors are seen as important but woolly. Perhaps the challenge to psychiatry should not be framed in terms of equal treatment. There is much evidence to suggest that 'equal treatment' in its most bland sense is precisely what has failed to reach those who are socially excluded, those in poverty as well as those from Black and minority ethnic groups. It is more differentiated treatment which is necessary, that is, the kind of person-centred approach that can accommodate the patient as an individual, and a patient's values and culture. It would be an approach that does not attempt to fit every patient into a diagnostic category signifying the same treatment for everyone, without regard for how patients themselves interpret their mental health. This is not simply a question of public relations where psychiatry is just 'misunderstood'. The onus is on psychiatrists to demonstrate greater sensitivity to the variation in explanatory models in mental health and the individual characteristics of the patient. This is the challenge of the practice problem.

Now, to the perception problem. There is no question that the causes of inequalities in the mental health system are not straightforward, and these are too complex to be covered here owing to lack of space. It is certain that psychiatrists are not responsible for all of them. However, some psychiatrists engage with these issues defensively and negatively, rather than as positively, or constructively, as they could. There is a problem with the way in which the mental health system is perceived among certain communities, but this should not distract us from the fact that there may be better, more comprehensive models of practice that could help psychiatrists communicate better with patients and would alleviate the perception of discrimination. In this way, changes in practice will drive changes in perception and bolster trust for psychiatrists.

If the approach of more psychiatrists were positive and constructive, psychiatric skills in this debate could be widely recognized as essential tools, and psychiatry would occupy its proper position as the leader of best practice, a lynchpin: demonstrating the ability to examine and coordinate new approaches to mental health right across the professions. This will require psychiatry to examine its problems honestly and debate them publicly, and to adopt wholeheartedly a more expansive understanding of how to create mental wellbeing rather than batten down the hatches and wait for the storm to pass. It won't.

What is psychiatry doing?

Some psychiatrists strive to introduce new paradigms. The Royal College of Psychiatrists has of course been very active in supporting cutting-edge developments in such areas as recovery, philosophy, and spirituality. It has also shown a very positive and inclusive approach to the critics of psychiatry, for example, through its inclusion of sessions and workshops organized by the Critical Psychiatry Network.

On a wider international front, the World Psychiatric Association launched a programme on 'Psychiatry for the Person', which covers diagnosis, models of disorder and public health as well as the more familiar areas of clinical training and service delivery, is precisely designed to bring the patient, as a unique individual, back to the focus of psychiatric care.

Bracken and his colleagues highlight what they call 'post-psychiatry', in which questions of social context, values and the patient's own model of the illness are central. The emphasis is taken off diagnostic pigeonholing without refuting the tools of traditional psychiatry. (Bracken 2001, 2002) challenges the assumption that psychiatric classification systems capture universal truths about distress and madness when they largely ignore the meaning the patient attaches to what he or she has experienced (Bracken, 2001, 2002). Similarly, the Critical Psychiatry Network promotes an ethical basis for the practice of psychiatry that places the concerns of service users, families, carer, and communities at the centre of their work (see Thomas & Bracken, 2004).

Another shift as a very practical application of the new philosophy of psychiatry has been the development of values-based practice, which has contributed to a number of national programmes over the last few years. Values-based practice brings a new approach to developing the skills-base that we need to integrate, the diverse resources for mental health from different disciplinary perspectives, and a strongly user-centred approach, that is sensitive to the diversity of individual strengths as well as needs.

A particular strength of values-based practice is the way that it helps to build the links between the skills of psychiatry and the skills of social care. This is a particularly exciting development because it aims to extend service user involvement from treatment to diagnosis, from service users 'having a say' in how they are treated, to 'having a say' also in how their problems are understood in the first place.

There are many examples of positive practice. However, if progress is to be made, psychiatrists themselves must seek to embed all this in everyday practice. Psychiatry has a choice: either to pursue an argument based on a narrow interpretation of what medicine is all about, defensively diagnosing; or to scan the horizon and get a broader perspective. Yet if it is the case that these new paradigms are discussed and accepted internally, this must be translated into practice, to change both the practice and the perception.

This would involve psychiatry seeing its place within the panoply of mental health services. It would involve acknowledging that psychiatric diagnosis cannot be divorced from the values both of the psychiatrist and the patient, and the decisions that each makes about treatment. It would involve considering how best to employ the skills of psychiatry in the interests of mental health service users.

Why are psychiatrists best placed to deliver a new approach?

For psychiatry to win back trust, it must accept that not all non-psychiatric models of mental illness are wrong. It must consider the 'politics of the patient'. This is not anti-psychiatrists or anti-psychiatry. In fact, this approach takes psychiatry back to its etymological roots as a 'healing of the soul', a definition which to me implies a more personalized response than any single medical model allows, and also a more expansive understanding of success about recovery and well-being rather than diagnosis or usage.

Science has a long and successful history of getting things wrong. Einstein changed our understanding of Newton's theory of mechanics, but that far from implies that Newton was a poor scientist. Part of science's success is in constant innovation and improvement: in new, better, more expansive ideas overtaking old ones that are found to be flawed in some respect.

One thing science never is, is stagnant. It is a discipline that by its nature is constantly developing. The idea that science shouldn't adapt, that it can find a 'right answer' and stick to it, is against what science stands for, and is fatally flawed.

Conclusions

Psychiatry is a science, and this applies. However, psychiatrists are not just scientists. They are also doctors, philosophers, advocates, guardians, therapists, and healers. The skills and disciplines that unite in psychiatry make psychiatrists uniquely placed to meet the challenges of the mental health system. The current climate can be seen as an opportunity rather than solely as a threat: and it should be more widely recognized that it is a threat only if psychiatry does not locate itself as the solution rather than the problem.

References

Bhui, K. S., & Bhugra, D. (2002). Mental illness in Black and Asian ethnic minorities: Pathways to care and outcomes. *Advances in Psychiatric Treatment,* **8**, 28–33.

Bhui, K. & Bhugra, D. (2002). Explanatory models for mental distress: implications for clinical practice and research (editorial). *British Journal of Psychiatry,* **181**, 6–7.

Bhui, K. S., Stansfeld, S., Hull, S., Priebe, S., Mole, F., & Feder, G. (2003). Ethnic variations in pathways to and use of specialist mental health services in the UK. *British Journal of Psychiatry,* **182**, 105–116.

Blomfield, A. (2007). Labelled mad for daring to criticise the Kremlin. *The Telegraph* 14 August, 2007. Retrieved 19 October 2007 from http://www.telegraph.co.uk/news/main.jhtml?xml=news/2007/08/13/wasylum113.xml

Bracken, P. (2001). Postpsychiatry: A new direction for mental health. *British Medical Journal,* **332**, 724–727.

Bracken, P. (2002). *Trauma: Culture, Meaning and Philosophy*. London: Whurr.

Commission for Healthcare Audit and Inspection. (2007). *Count Me in Census*. London: Department of Health.

Department of Health, Inside Outside: Improving mental health services for black and minority ethnic communities in England, 2003.

Foucault, M. (2001). *Madness and Civilization*. London: Routledge (trans Richard Howard).

Ipsos-MORI . (2005). Science in Society: Findings from Qualitative Research (13). A Report Conducted for the Office of Science and Technology, Department of Trade and Industry.

Mental Health Foundation. (2006). *We Need to Talk: The Case for Psychological Therapy on the NHS*. London: Mental Health Foundation.

Muller, H. J. 1890-167, Science and Criticism (1943).

Norfolk, Suffolk and Cambridgeshire Strategic Health Authority, Independent Inquiry into the death of David Bennett, 2003.

Royal College of Psychiatrists. (2006). *College Response to the Health Select Committee Enquiry into Workforce Needs and Planning*. London: Royal College of Psychiatrists.

Sieghart, P. (1985). Professions as the conscience of society. *Journal of Medical Ethics*, **11**, 117–122.

The Sainsbury Centre for Mental Health, Breaking the *Circles of Fear*, 2002.

Thomas, P., & Bracken, P. (2004). Critical psychiatry in practice. *Advances in Psychiatric Treatment*, **10**, 361–370.

YouGov (2007). Poll Commissioned by Mental Health Charity Rethink.

Chapter 5

Economics and society: efficiency, equity, and choice

Paul Freddolino and Martin Knapp

Introduction

Trying to determine the best psychiatric practice has become at the same time both more challenging and more feasible with the tremendous range of resources available in contemporary practice. With a growing number of journals reporting studies of relevance to psychiatric practice as well as numerous syntheses of individual studies such as those by the Cochrane Collaboration, the resources are both invaluable and daunting. Even attempts to codify the results of these studies into usable tools such as the 13 American Psychiatric Association's practice guidelines (American Psychiatric Association, 2006) and the clinical guidelines prepared by the National Institute for Health and Clinical Excellence in England and Wales (2008) present valuable insights and perhaps even too much information.

Although there is no legal requirement for psychiatrists and other health professionals to use 'evidence-based' or 'best' medical practice, ethical guidelines have moved beyond the Hippocratic injunction to 'do no harm' to positive statements encouraging physicians to maximize health for individual patients. In the United Kingdom, the *Guidelines for Good Medical Practice* state that doctors must 'provide a good standard of practice and care' based on keeping their 'professional knowledge and skills up to date'(General Medical Council, 2006). In the United States, the American Medical Association notes in its *Principles of Medical Ethics* (American Medical Association, 2001) that physicians shall 'continue to study, apply, and advance scientific knowledge' and be 'dedicated to providing competent medical care'. In its *Principles of Medical Ethics with Annotations Especially Applicable to Psychiatry* (American Psychiatric Association, 2009) the American Psychiatric Association notes that 'a psychiatrist's treatment plan shall be based on clinical, scientific, or generally accepted standards of treatment'. The World Medical Association (WMA) International Code of Medical Ethics (2006) states that a physician 'shall owe his/her patients complete loyalty and all the scientific resources available to him/her'.

When we move beyond the level of the individual patient to a collective level, however, additional factors demand consideration. The WMA (2006) notes that physicians 'shall strive to use health care resources in the best way to benefit patients and their community', raising the question of what criteria need to be considered in the determination of what is 'best'. There are many candidate criteria but in this chapter we concentrate on three of the most important factors, each of which is particularly associated with the economics literature: efficiency, equity, and choice. *Efficiency* refers to the relationship between resources used up and changes achieved as a result. In particular, the pursuit of efficiency is to search for ways to spend available budgets or to deploy available services so as to achieve the maximum effects in terms of good outcomes for patients (linked to, for example, meeting needs, alleviating symptoms, or improving quality of life). *Equity*, on the other hand, refers to the distribution of those resources and the distribution of their effects. In particular, the equity criterion seeks to ensure that access to services, responsibility for payment for them, and the health and quality of life outcomes that result are allocated or distributed fairly across the population. A third criterion for determining what is the 'best' or a 'better' way to use health care resources is *choice*, a value embedded in many (particularly Western) societies and an outcome consistent with the ethical principles of informed patient consent and the competent patient's right to accept or refuse treatment.

In this chapter we will examine the relevance of each of these three criteria in decision making with respect to mental health treatment, support, and promotion. We consider the barriers that make implementation of these criteria in decision making problematic and how these barriers might be addressed. We conclude with suggestions for future research and the involvement of the psychiatric community in moving the quality of psychiatric treatment decision-making forward. We should also emphasize at the outset that the three criteria of efficiency, equity, and choice are not independent of one another although initially we discuss them separately.

Efficiency

In every mental health system across the world, it is recognized that there will never be enough resources to meet all mental health needs, whether those are the expressed or diagnosed needs of people already in contact with the system, or the underlying and partly unrecognized needs of the population. Given this pervasive scarcity, careful choices must be made about how to make best use of what is available. For example, should there be greater investment in the training and deployment of clinical psychologists or a bigger budget for medications? What proportion of a mental health budget should be allocated, not for the treatment of identified needs but instead to uncover previously unrecognized needs? What resources should be devoted to mental health promotion, seeking to prevent problems from emerging in the first place? When does it make sense to reduce the intensity of treatment for one particular patient and to use the time to initiate a treatment programme for someone who has been newly referred?

None of these questions is first and foremost *economic* in nature, but each stems from recognition of the scarcity of resources relative to needs, and so each generates questions about what resources get used and with what consequences, and it is those latter questions that certainly have an economic flavour. In fact, each of those latter questions concerns the relationship between the budgets needed or expended, the services or support arrangements provided as a result, and the outcomes that are achieved for individuals, families, and the wider society (Knapp & McDaid, 2007).

Consequently, anyone with any responsibility for deciding on the use of resources (budgets, services, staff time, medications) needs to be clear about the basis on which he or she chooses one option over another. One of the criteria likely to be used to inform such decisions is efficiency, which means achieving the maximum effects in terms of services delivered or outcomes achieved, such as needs met, symptoms alleviated, or quality of life improved, from a specified volume of resources such as an available budget or a fixed number of therapy sessions per week. The fragmented nature of most mental health systems, with multiple sources of funding and multiple service delivery and support mechanisms – from health, social care, housing, criminal justice, and other systems – can make it hard to pursue efficiency if insufficient attention is paid to coordination and cooperation. This proved particularly important, for example, when the balance of care was shifting from hospital-dominated to community-orientated mental health treatment and support. There is also the growing reliance on multi-professional teams, liaison services, 'whole systems' approaches, and so on. In each case, inter- and intra-agency rivalries, administrative bureaucracy, and a desire to protect existing budgets may mean that society's scarce resources will continue to be used in a manner that reflects interests (defensible or otherwise) other than efficiency.

The influence of the efficiency criterion can be seen in many decision-making spheres. Commissioners who are locally responsible for purchasing services to meet the needs of their local populations want to get the best they can in terms of improved patient health from their limited budgets. Companies that sell medications or other 'health technologies' often employ both effectiveness and cost-effectiveness evidence in their marketing efforts. (We define cost-effectiveness in a moment.) Bodies charged with technology appraisal and/or with advising on the take-up of treatments (such as the National Institute for Health and Clinical Excellence [NICE] in England and Wales) similarly want evidence on efficiency: does this particular treatment represent good 'value for money' for the health system? Policymakers at a central level certainly want to be sure that the resources for which they are responsible are used to best effect; furthermore, agencies charged with monitoring and regulation (such as the Care Quality Commission in England) also have this interest in mind.

The efficiency analysis most commonly discussed in the mental health field is cost-effectiveness analysis. It is a form of analysis particularly designed to pool information on both the costs (resources employed) and the effectiveness (outcomes) of two or more treatments or support options. The central question asked by a cost-effectiveness analysis is whether the improved outcomes from one intervention over another are *worth* the extra cost of achieving them. Deciding what outcome is or is not 'worth' the cost is far from straightforward but is the very crux of an economic evaluation (see, for example, Knapp & Beecham, 2009).

Although across the world even private psychiatric practices operate in the very public world of insurance, government allocations, and limitations on consumer resources, very little time is devoted to health economics in general or efficiency in particular in the everyday activities of psychiatrists. We are not arguing that every decision taken by a psychiatrist needs to be filtered through an efficiency check, not the least because there are many other relevant criteria to be taken into account (including the other two criteria – equity and choice – discussed below). However, it behoves psychiatrists to avoid the unnecessary waste of resources. If two courses of action – say two treatment approaches – are identical in their effects on patient health and are equally acceptable to those patients, it would not make sense to choose the one that is more expensive. Part of psychiatry's contract with society is to contribute to the more efficient use of available resources – to recognize not just the pertinence but the imperative of cost-effectiveness – for in this way, the constrained resources allocated to a mental health system can have greater aggregate impact on individual and societal well-being.

Equity

All mental health systems are inherently if not necessarily deliberately inequitable. They do not distribute the benefits of treatment and support or the burdens of paying for them fairly across the population. Instead – wittingly or unwittingly – they allow demographic, cultural, social, economic, or political considerations to have an influence. As a result, access to, impact of, or payment for treatment is unfairly distributed by gender, ethnicity, age, language, religion, income, socioeconomic group, or the place of residence.

However, what do 'fair' and 'unfair' mean? It would be seen by most people as unfair if everyone in the population had exactly the same amount of support or treatment from the mental health system because many people have no need for any such support at all, whereas a few people have very considerable needs. Making sure everyone had an equal *right* or *access* to treatment when they were ill might be thought to be fair(er). An equitable allocation of mental health resources would also usually mean giving more treatment or support to people with greater needs, whereas an equitable approach to the *financing* of a health system would usually mean ensuring that those people with the least ability to pay for their treatment (generally those with lower incomes) are charged lower amounts than those with greater ability to pay (higher incomes). Consequently, in broad terms the two most commonly discussed aspects of equity are as follows:

1 Whether individual financial contributions are linked to ability to pay and whether there should be a redistributive effort so that low-income individuals contribute proportionately lower amounts; and

2 whether access to evidence-based treatment is linked to type, urgency, and severity of need and not to ability to pay.

Every mental health system across the world is inequitable to some degree, and of course there are gross inequities *between* such systems given the huge disparities across the globe in the availability of skilled health care (Saxena, Thornicroft, Knapp, & Whiteford, 2007). In countries that rely heavily on private insurance funding mechanisms such as the United States, the poor have worse access and get worse treatment than the rich (U.S. Department of Health and Human Services, 1999). The National Health Service in the United Kingdom is more egalitarian in intent, with its universal coverage and with its financing based on a tax system that is generally held to be progressive and redistributive (hence addressing in part the first aspect of equity distinguished above). Even so, there still appear to be some links between socioeconomic position, prevalence, and treatment (Mangalore, Knapp, & Jenkins, 2007) as well as alarmingly wide disparities in the experiences of people from different ethnic groups in terms of the kinds of treatment they are offered and actually experience (McKenzie & Bhui, 2007; McKenzie et al., 2001).

There is also evidence of age discrimination in the United Kingdom. New statistical analyses, supported by the views of people interviewed in mental health organizations, show that use of mental health services is lower among older people, even after adjusting for symptoms and need (Beecham et al., 2008).

The age gradient in service use appears to be more marked for 'common mental disorders' such as depression and anxiety than for more severe mental health problems. Indeed, for people with psychosis there may be an increase in health service use beyond about age 60 although whether this is mainly in the use of general health services rather than mental health services is not clear. Some but not all analyses suggest that the age gradient is more marked for men than for women.

Another major concern – worldwide – is the stigma widely associated with mental illness (Schomerus & Angermeyer, 2008). Individuals may be fearful of discrimination if they are labelled as having a mental health problem (Corrigan & Wassel, 2008). Inequity in this case may be especially marked in relation to, for example, access to paid employment and other forms of social participation. Compared to people with other health needs, people with mental health issues fare badly, contributing considerably to social exclusion (Social Exclusion Unit, 2004).

The actions of individual psychiatrists cannot, alone, make much of a difference to the distributional characteristics of a health system, but they can make an enormous difference to the perceived fairness of the treatment (or the experiences more generally) of individual patients. Of course, the accumulated actions of many psychiatrists can be quite noticeable, so that if there is a widespread if individually generated tendency for bias to the disadvantage of older people (say), the aggregate effect could be significant. Highly trained professionals such as psychiatrists, necessarily working in one-to-one relationships with patients, should be aware of the cumulative consequences of their decisions. They should also be aware of the cumulative *power* of their reporting of underserved needs and their lobbying for greater equity. (This is recognized in, for example, the AMA's statement VII (2001): 'A physician shall recognize a responsibility to participate in activities contributing to the improvement of the community and the betterment of public health'.) Moreover, psychiatrists in senior administrative and decision-making positions are better placed to exert an influence.

Part of any contract with society must be a commitment to agreed social mores and to socially agreed priorities (where they exist or can be discerned, of course) to the fairer allocation of psychiatric and other health services, and to socially agreed principles of equity more generally. Those principles might not get discussed by reference to any particular theoretical precepts (such as the well-known Rawlsian 'maximin' principles (Rawls, 1973) or Sen's capabilities approach (Sen, 1999)), but most governments of the world and the United Nations through three of its eight Millenium Development Goals have policies aimed at improving fairness, whether through their tax system, through their support for particular models of health financing, or through their commitment to eradicate disparities linked to ethnicity, gender, or age.

Choice

Choice is central to classical economic thought: freedom of choice (backed up by the wherewithal to express that freedom in the marketplace) ensures that producers of goods and services deliver what consumers actually want and at a price they are willing to pay. Free choice promotes competition, which works to improve the quality of products, to keep prices down, and to ensure that scarce resources are employed in the production of goods and services that maximize the well-being of citizens. In this way, choice can improve the efficiency of the economy. It might not do much to enhance equity except insofar as the protection or promotion of individual rights to realistic self-determination is itself an objective with equity overtones. So far, so Adam Smith.

However, even Adam Smith recognized that freely functioning markets were more of an ideal or an aspiration than a reality. However, mental health services are not like groceries. Individuals needing food use their own income to purchase groceries. The store owner purchases stocks of groceries from a wholesaler, and then through various links in the economic chain the funds reach the farmers who grow or rear the ingredients. At each stage the purchaser (including the ultimate consumer) has the freedom to decide whether to make the purchase, primarily based on their assessment of product quality and price. If the quality is insufficient to justify the price, they will go elsewhere until they have found a product that is worth buying. In this way, the simple workings of a market economy generally function well enough to allocate groceries to people who want them and have the money to buy them. There can be glitches, but the usual way to overcome them is to make some adjustment to market forces, including providing subsidies to poorer consumers, for example, through food vouchers or social security payments.

Of course, mental health services differ from groceries in many and profound ways, not least because they are much more complex products. It is relatively straightforward for a consumer to ascertain the quality of groceries, but it is much harder for a mental health service user to judge the quality of potential treatments. Although individuals usually have a fairly clear idea of the groceries they need, people with mental health needs will often have only limited knowledge of the treatments available, how they might meet their needs, and with what side-effects. The stigma and prejudice that continue to surround mental health services may also mean that some people are unwilling or too embarrassed to be seen to purchase products that would help them.

For these and other reasons it is widely recognized that a mental health system cannot be constructed along simple unfettered, unregulated market lines emphasizing individual choice if it is to be efficient and equitable. Not only are mental health services inherently complex products, but most people who need or use them are not experienced consumers with access to the available evidence base that would allow them to decide what is good or bad, suitable or unsuitable.

However, although 'textbook markets' may not be suitable for a mental health system, there are nevertheless many reasons to advocate giving people greater choice and control over the services and treatments they need and are offered. Social work and other professions have long emphasized independence and empowerment, thereby giving normative professional credibility to devolved commissioning powers. The WMA (2006) notes that physicians shall 'respect the rights and preferences of patients,' and even the American Psychiatric Association notes that psychiatrists shall 'make relevant information available to patients, colleagues, and the public' (APA, 2009, p. 10), although this principle is not followed with specific guidance for how it should be done.

The encouragement of informed individual choice appeals both to the political Right because of its links to market mechanisms, and also to the Centre Left because of its connections with citizenship, participation, and accountability in public services. Certain kinds of arrangement might also be seen to be sympathetic towards community development ideologies on the Left. From the user perspective, greater powers of choice and control can be attractive because of the empowerment offered and are clearly supportive of rights-based agenda. An NIMHE booklet (Glasby et al., 2003) identified five reasons for involving service users and the general public in decision making: accountability, developing local understanding, strengthening public confidence, encouraging services to become more responsive, and challenging any paternalistic models of provision. User involvement brings a particular expertise and a different perspective to the decision-making forum; it can be therapeutic; and it can help new approaches to meeting needs to emerge.

Consequently, policies aimed at extending choice in public services (sometimes called 'personalization' in health and social care contexts in the United Kingdom) appeal to many different groups and agenda. This does not mean that they are problem-free, especially when it comes to the tricky issue of balancing empowerment with safeguarding. Moreover, not every individual user of mental health services will have the competence, confidence, or desire to take responsibility for how the public or other funds are spent on their care. Even with very good brokerage, and care management more generally, individual and personal budgets might not be sensible for everyone.

Another important reality that is pushing the issue of choice into a position of greater prominence than previously is the absolute explosion of information – ranging from the accurate to the absolutely dangerous – available through the Internet (Psych Central, 2010). Although, as noted above, at the point of contact with a psychiatrist an individual may have limited awareness of effective alternatives and limited competence to make such decisions, once that moment has passed he or she, together with significant others and mental health advocates of all stripes, will have access to a wide range of fact and opinion concerning diagnoses, prognoses, and possible treatments. Thus very quickly the encounter between psychiatrist and patient can turn from having limited knowledge at hand to having voluminous information that must be evaluated, digested, and ultimately prioritized in the context of the specific patient's situation.

What does this imply for psychiatry's contract with society? The American Psychiatric Association clearly indicates that 'psychiatrists are responsible for their own continuing education and should be mindful of the fact that theirs must be a lifetime of learning' (APA, 2009, p. 10). Taken together with the previously noted injunction to make relevant information available to patients, colleagues, and the public, and the simple reality that patients have incredibly enhanced access to information – not all of it accurate – the guidance from the profession seems to suggest the necessity of a greater educational role for psychiatry than in previous periods. At the level of individual practitioners this will mean remaining up to date with the latest research findings relevant to treatments for the types of patients they regularly encounter. It is only in this way that practitioners can provide information that will support the informed decision and consent of their patients as soon as adequate competence to decide is reached. At the collective level it will mean evaluating and highlighting reputable sources of information for patients, their family and friends, other mental health professionals, and the public to turn to in their search for accurate information.

To the extent that truly informed choice will have an impact both on efficiency and equity in mental health services, this aspect of the contract with society may in fact be the most pressing. However, to carry out this educational role there will be greater dependence on the types of information that economists and other evaluation professionals generate, information that has in the past encountered serious barriers to recognition and acceptance by psychiatry. Understanding these barriers and how they might be overcome is the ultimate intent of this chapter, and the topic to which we now turn.

Barriers

Despite the various guidelines and good practice standards from, for example, the World Medical Association and professional groups in the United Kingdom, United States, and elsewhere supporting the use of evaluative research that can enhance the achievement of efficiency, equity, and choice in the mental health arena, it is clear that such research is not used effectively in contemporary psychiatric practice. The reasons for the failure of evaluative perspectives to gain traction are numerous and can be divided into three general areas: (1) issues related to the quality of the research process and research studies; (2) what might be called 'professional' issues; and (3) ethical, political, and value debates.

Research issues

The relatively low rate of implementation by decision makers of recommendations stemming from efficiency, equity, and choice studies seems, on the one hand, to reflect barriers to potentially relevant evaluative evidence rather than resistance to the criteria themselves. Frankly, even when considering only clinical trials sponsored by industry under strict government regulations or conducted by academic institutions under government research grants, there is a minimum amount of clinically relevant evidence (Geddes, 2005). Furthermore, there are several characteristics of the evaluative literature that contribute to the perception of inadequacy of the research evidence base and thus erode its potential usefulness and impact.

There is inadequate evidence to address many real-world questions and concerns of psychiatrists and their patients. Despite improvements in the past decade, the body of research from which many conclusions are drawn has not included adequate studies of the effects – both positive and harmful – on various age, gender, and ethnic groups, and thus may not recognize the different effects that the same treatment may have on different people under different circumstances. We are a long way from having evaluative studies that can tell us what treatments work best with what types of patients under what conditions and at what costs.

In areas where there has been a greater volume of research and evaluation, multiple studies frequently lead to contradictory findings and ever-changing conclusions. This raises a concern about what indeed is actually known or can be concluded about the absolute and relative efficacy, efficiency, and equity implications of various treatments.

There are important outcome measurement issues including the lack of agreement on what outcomes are meaningful for various subject populations, and the failure of researchers to agree how the outcomes should be measured to be considered scientifically valid (Jacobs & McDaid, 2009). For example, what does good 'quality of life' mean for patients who differ by race, age, or ethnicity, and how should it be measured? In addition there is concern that considerable funding from large pharmaceutical companies to support outcome research studies inherently creates conflicts of interest and raises questions about the quality and integrity of research findings.

Finally, there are major gaps in the communication of relevant findings to psychiatrists and the public. This is further complicated by the often tremendous time lag from the conduct of research in laboratory or controlled conditions to actual experience with the treatment by patients. This inevitably leads to suspicions as to whether the findings actually reflect what will *really* be the effects of treatments.

Although some of the opposition to evaluative perspectives can thus be attributed to characteristics of the relevant research literature, additional barriers can be attributed to what might be called professional resistance to the value of such research studies. Furthermore, broader public debate concerning the notion that cost should limit personal and professional choice in treatment, and concerning the relative 'value' of different treatment scenarios, adds to the hurdles confronting utilization of economics research findings.

Professional issues

Psychiatry is not alone among the professions or even among medical specialties in raising questions about the value, usefulness, and even appropriateness of rigorous economic and other evaluation research studies. Four concerns are frequently raised by these professional groups.

Perhaps the most fundamental concern involves a more influential role – perhaps even a definitive role – for government-funded or government-sanctioned outcomes research that will mean putting government agencies directly in the middle of the doctor–patient relationship, something seen as harmful for a wide range of reasons. This is a concern much more frequently expressed in the United States than in the United Kingdom, but it is or should be an important consideration in every society and system.

The second concern focuses on the nature of psychiatric crises. There is considerable anecdotal evidence that in times of psychiatric crisis, both patients and their families want to know about one or two choices, described by a trusted psychiatrist, together with a professional recommendation as to which one would be 'best' for the patient. This is particularly the case in the face of multiple potential interventions that have been evaluated through a set of 'inconclusive' research studies that can be accessed by families and other patient advocates. This does not mean that patient choice is or ever should be anathema in a mental health context, for there are all kinds of advance directives and proxy arrangements that can be put into place, but it does mean that the context for extending choice differs somewhat from what would apply in many other areas of health or social care. In particular, a careful balance will also need to be struck between safeguarding and empowerment.

Third, there is generalized professional resistance among psychiatrists to non-psychiatrists having the ultimate decision-making role in treatment decisions. Ultimately, many psychiatrists believe that non-psychiatrists simply do not understand the complexities of diagnosis and treatment. This professional bias is not unique to psychiatry, but its presence there affects the broader mental health services arena.

Finally, there is the concern that the underlying commitment to the uniqueness of each patient long held as sacrosanct by psychiatry will be undermined by 'formulae' based on 'reductionist research' as to which treatment must be prescribed for all patients with a certain diagnosis. There is a thin line between guideline and directive, whether in actuality or in professional perception.

The great debates

The types of debates heard in the United States in 2009 reflect those heard in the past – and in fact still heard – in other parts of the world. These are debates about core values and beliefs – deeply held, slow to change. They cover a wide range of ethical and political issues, many of which reflect differences about underlying values concerning access to health care and definitions of 'health' and 'quality of life'.

Despite a growing awareness in many societies that there are limits to the amount of money that can or should be spent on medical care, there is tremendous disagreement over whether *cost* should be a factor in making individual patient decisions. Fears include arbitrary rationing of mental health and other care as well as the realistic potential for greater inequity in distribution of the inevitably limited resources. If cost is to be considered, there will obviously be a role for economic evaluation research.

There is considerable disagreement about the 'value' of alternative outcomes for a fixed amount of public expenditure; for example, do we use funds to treat a larger number of mildly ill people, or spend that same amount but on a smaller number of people with more serious symptoms? Should treating one person with schizophrenia be considered the same as treating one person with dementia? In the absence of answers to such questions – in other words, on the trade-offs that society considers to be appropriate – it is very difficult for some types of economic evaluation research to make progress in its acceptance to psychiatry and to other communities because the bases of outcome measurement and weighting will always be challenged.

What should be the role of pharmaceutical companies in these debates? The extensive advertising seen on television, in magazines, and on the Internet (although varying by country) indicates that there are numerous financial outcomes at stake. This raises the importance of asking to what extent 'educational' efforts by pharmaceutical companies are in reality marketing efforts targeted at each drug-appropriate market.

There is considerable potential use for evaluative evidence in meeting the spirit of good practice in psychiatry suggested by various guidelines based on the criteria of efficiency, equity, and choice. However, all of the issues noted above create barriers to the utilization of findings from even the very best evaluative research studies conducted by the most reputable researchers under the most stringent research criteria. Some resolution of this dilemma would add value to contemporary psychiatry's contract with society, and we will share some possible paths forward in the concluding section.

Conclusion

A decade ago one of us reviewed the state of the art in economic evaluation and concluded as follows:

> Although the number and sophistication of economic evaluations have both increased noticeably over recent years, there remain imbalances. . . . Many challenges consequently face the next generation of mental health economics evaluations, both for research economists and for those health care decision-makers who find themselves increasingly having to draw on economics evidence (Knapp, 1999, p.163).

A review of developments in the subsequent decade would surely conclude that many of the same challenges remain at a time when fiscal constraints will force even more attention onto costs (especially with public debt escalating in the face of the worldwide financial crisis) leading to more pressure to use evaluative results and a lower willingness to pay for treatments solely on the basis of 'faith', 'hunch', or anecdote.

There is a lot of blame to go around in the search for scapegoats. As noted above, there is clear evidence of both the failure of economists and other evaluative researchers to produce high-quality studies that address the types of real-world questions faced by psychiatrists, patients, families, and those who pay for treatments and services. At the same time, resistance to the evaluation enterprise by professionals, patients, and the public unwilling to face some fiscal realities and moral dilemmas undercuts the value of the good evaluative studies that have been completed.

Ultimately the solution may require a higher degree of collaboration between psychiatrists and other professionals, including researchers – collaboration done carefully, thoughtfully, and consistent with psychiatric values – but nevertheless undertaken as a serious and valuable enterprise. For example, to improve the quality of the evaluative research available to psychiatrists, practitioners must get more involved in the research process. They know the types of practical questions that must be faced in emergency situations and thus can help design studies that provide more complete and realistic analyses. Psychiatry's insistence on the need to improve the quality of research will be perceived as more genuine if the critique comes with the offer to participate in the research process. In that way, psychiatrists can have a constructive influence on the formation and execution of the evaluative studies.

A second area where collaboration is required is in the area of funding for high-quality evaluative research. Psychiatrists need to push for additional funding from independent sources to support the extensive amount of robust research still required. In this effort, funding from pharmaceutical companies must be balanced with funding from elsewhere to reduce complaints about the objectivity of evidence. Despite some aversion to funding from governmental bodies in some quarters (again, more of an issue in the United States than the United Kingdom), this source will become increasingly important as it becomes clear to public bodies how much of their funding can be saved (or, better still, utilized more efficiently in other ways) by building on evidence-based practices.

A third area for collaboration is related to the communication flow of new information in usable form from evaluative researchers both to psychiatrists and then from psychiatrists to patients and the general public (as well as, of course, directly to patients, families, and others). Joint efforts in research should lead to joint strategies in communicating the results of the studies to multiple audiences. There is also a need to make sure that communication runs in the other direction, from the potential and actual 'subjects' of research to those who commission and conduct studies. Professional associations in psychiatry should ensure that new psychiatrists are trained in how to locate and utilize the results of the best studies to decrease the lag time into practice. Psychiatrists with the wisdom of practice experience should participate in constructive ways in discussions about research findings that advance the ultimate understanding of research results for the practice area in question. These psychiatrists should also play an active role in communicating to patients, families, and the public the evolving understanding of what practices are in fact the *best practices* for specific conditions.

However, this is not sufficient, for there is also surely an obligation to play active roles in research that addresses other, generally broader societal concerns of the kind discussed in this chapter. To be meaningful and effective in the twenty-first century, psychiatry's contract with society should include supporting endeavours – through research, lobbying, and action – to improve the efficiency with which available resources are used (including psychiatrists' own time), to achieve more equitable allocations of benefits and burdens, and to create appropriate opportunities for patients to exercise meaningful choice. At the same time, it must be acknowledged that these three goals may have to be pursued along parallel tracks given their complexity, even though a look at the range of 'best practice' choices available to patients in various income and gender groups clearly demonstrates the reality that these three criteria are not independent of one another.

This chapter began with references to the voluminous information, evaluative study results, and other resources in the mental health arena available to patients, families, governments, and the public. There is a clear demand by patients and other stakeholders for assistance in identifying compact solutions to this information overload, and psychiatry's absence from the effort to improve the quality and the usefulness of this information will not make either the amount of information or the demand for clarity disappear. Any reluctance on psychiatry's part to engage on this issue will only provide an opportunity for others – frequently less expert – to fill the void. In mental health as in other fields, information and how it is shaped and made available becomes a great source of power and influence, and for the good of both society and the psychiatric profession, it is important that psychiatry's twenty-first century contract includes a meaningful role in this effort.

References

American Medical Association. (2001). AMA Code of Medical Ethics: Principles of Medical Ethics. Retrieved 3 June 2009 from http://www.ama-assn.org/ama/pub/physician-resources/medical-ethics/code-medical-ethics/principles-medical-ethics.shtml .

American Psychiatric Association. (2006). *American Psychiatric Association Practice Guidelines for the Treatment of Psychiatric Disorders: Compendium 2006.* American Psychiatric Publishing.

American Psychiatric Association. (2009). *The Principles of Medical Ethics with Annotations Especially Applicable to Psychiatry.* Virginia: American Psychiatric Association.

Beecham, J., Knapp, M., Fernandez, L J., et al. (2008). Age discrimination in mental health services. PSSRU Discussion Paper. London School of Economics and Political Science.

Corrigan, P. W., & Wassel, A. (2008). Understanding and influencing the stigma of mental illness. *Journal of Psychosocial Nursing and Mental Health Services,* 46, 42–48.

Geddes, J. R. (2005). Large simple trials in psychiatry: Providing reliable answers to important clinical questions. *Epidemiologia e Psichiatria Sociale,* 14, 122–126.

General Medical Council. (2006). Good Medical Practice. Retrieved 3 June 2009 from http://www.gmc-uk.org/guidance/good_medical_practice/duties_of_a_doctor.asp.

Glasby, J., Lester, H., Briscoe, J., Clark, M., Rose, S., & England, L. (2003). *Cases for Change: User Involvement.* London: Department of Health/National Institute for Mental Health.

Jacobs, R., & McDaid, D. (2009). Performance assessment in mental health services. In P. Smith, E. Mossialos, S. Leatherman, & I. Papanicolas (Eds), *Performance Measurement for Health System Improvement: Experiences, Challenges and Prospects* (pp. 426–471). Cambridge: Cambridge University Press.

Knapp, M. (1999). Economic evaluation and mental health: Sparse past... fertile future? *Journal of Mental Health Policy and Economics,* **2,** 163–167.

Knapp, M., & Beecham, J. (2009). Health economics and psychiatry: The pursuit of efficiency. In D. Bhugra, & C. Morgan (Eds), *Principles of Social Psychiatry* (2nd ed) (pp. 549–561). Oxford: Blackwell Scientific Publications.

Knapp, M., & McDaid, D. (2007). Financing and funding mental health care services. In M. Knapp, D. McDaid, E. Mossialos, & G. Thornicroft (Eds), *Mental Health Policy and Practice across Europe* (pp. 60–99). Buckingham: Open University Press.

Mangalore, R., Knapp, M., & Jenkins, R. (2007). Income-related inequality in mental health in Britain: The concentration index approach. *Psychological Medicine,* **37,** 1037–1046.

McKenzie, K., & Bhui, K. (2007). Institutional racism in mental health care. *British Medical Journal,* **334,** 649–650.

McKenzie, K., Samele, C., van Horn, E., Tattan, T., van Os, J., & Murray, R. M. (2001). A comparison of the course and treatment of psychosis in patients of Caribbean origin and British whites. *British Journal of Psychiatry,* **178,** 160–165.

National Institute for Health and Clinical Excellence. (2008). Clinical Guidelines. Retrieved 3 June 2009 from http://www.nice.org.uk/guidance/CG.

Psych Central. (2010). *Mental Health and Psychology Resources Online.* Retrieved 24 August 2010 from http://psychcentral.com/resources/

Rawls, J. (1973). *A Theory of Justice.* Oxford: Oxford University Press.

Saxena, S., Thornicroft, G., Knapp, M., & Whiteford, H. (2007). Scarcity, inequity and inefficiency of resources: Three major obstacles to better mental health. *Lancet,* **370,** 878–889.

Schomerus, G., & Angermeyer, M. C. (2008). Stigma and its impact on help seeking for mental disorders: What do we know? *Epidemiologia e Psichiatria Sociale,* **7,** 31–37.

Sen, A. (1999). *Development as Freedom.* Oxford: Oxford University Press.

Social Exclusion Unit. (2004). *Mental Health and Social Exclusion.* London: Office of the Deputy Prime Minister.

The World Medical Association. (2006). World Medical Association International Code of Medical Ethics: Duties of Physicians in General. Retrieved 3 June 2009 from http://www.wma.net/e/policy/c8.htm

U.S. Department of Health and Human Services. (1999). *Mental Health: A Report of the Surgeon General.* Rockville, MD: U.S. Department of Health and Human Services, Substance Abuse and Mental Health Services Administration, Center for Mental Health Services, National Institutes of Health, National Institute of Mental Health.

Chapter 6

Stakeholders' expectations of psychiatric professionalism

Dinesh Bhugra, Susham Gupta, Genevieve Smyth, and Martin Webber

Introduction

Although it is an individual who suffers from a mental illness, it is inevitable that those around the said individual will be affected at a number of levels. Those who care for the person with a mental illness, those members of kinship and society who may have indirect contact with the individual, and the carers will influence the treatment and the therapeutic alliance. Once the individual develops symptoms of mental illness, and these symptoms are identified and realized to be abnormal either by the individual himself/herself or by the family members, it may be decided to seek therapeutic intervention. Depending upon how they perceive these abnormalities, that is, what their explanations are, whether they see these as caused by supra-natural, natural, social, psychological, or medical factors, they may seek help accordingly. The resources they have and the health care system locally available and, its accessibility will dictate the source they seek help from. In some settings a vast majority of patients with mental illness will be treated in folk or social sectors and will not reach the 'professional' sector simply because the latter may not be geographically and emotionally accessible. Once these obstacles have been dealt with, the individual with symptoms may see a professional, either a general practitioner or a specialist through the general practitioner or directly. Thereafter a series of factors come into play to reach a level of therapeutic alliance and treatment adherence. The therapeutic relationship between the patient and the psychiatrist will inevitably be influenced by a number of external factors.

Depending upon cultures and societies at a macro level, and symptoms, expectations of treatment and outcomes at a micro level, the therapeutic interaction will work at different levels.

Embedded within the consultation are two key individuals – the person who may see himself or herself as having an illness or sickness and the person he or she has come to see to get some treatment. Each of them brings to the therapeutic encounter personal factors such as age, gender, culture, and educational and socioeconomic status. Each of these factors will influence the explanatory model of the symptoms, which will also be affected by a number of other factors such as previous experience of illness and carers' explanatory models and training and clinical experience of the clinician.

The therapeutic interaction will also be influenced by what stage the help is sought at and explanatory models used (see Figure 6.1).

Therapeutic encounters can be roughly defined as a meeting of the individual with psychiatric symptoms who has not yet 'become' a patient and the clinician (in this case a psychiatrist) to understand the patient's experience and distress, and attempts to alleviate it using a number of strategies and techniques. Such an encounter is shown in Figure 6.2.

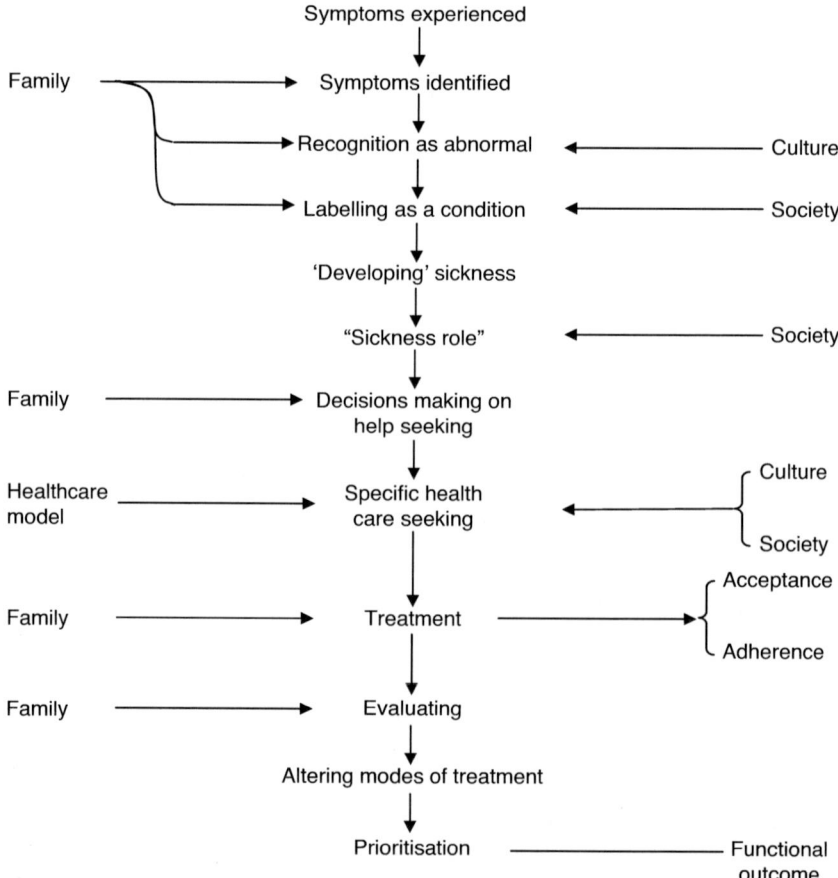

Fig. 6.1 Development of symptoms and external factors

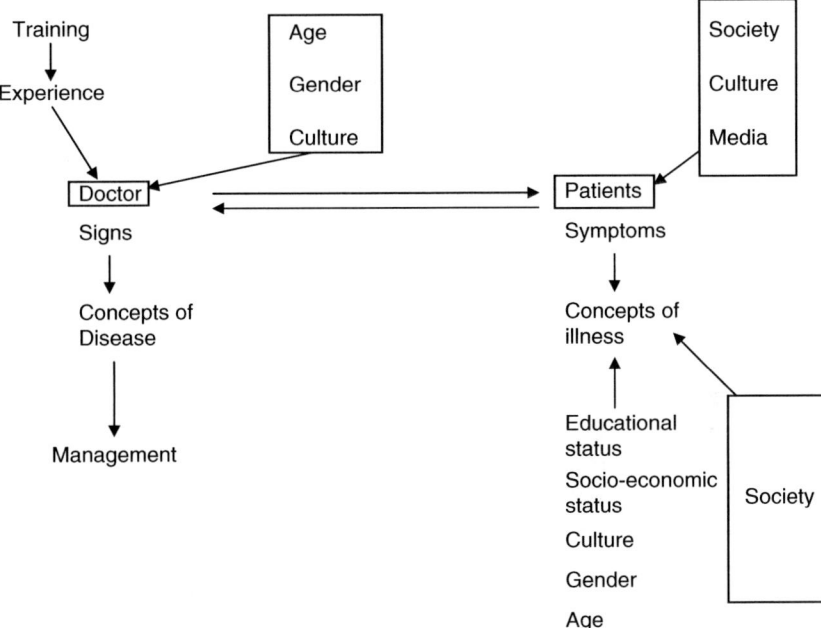

Fig. 6.2 Some factors in the therapeutic encounter

Expectations

Patients' and their carers' expectations can be broadly divided into those related to the therapeutic encounter (i.e., the process) and those related to the psychiatrist (i.e., the attitude) and the system. Sometimes both of these get muddled. It is important that when a clinician attempts to look at these it is clear as to what is being explored. Satisfaction from services may be dependent upon more superficial issues such as décor of the consultation room or the ward and access to private facilities, but the components of therapeutic interaction may remain untapped in any such assessment. When asking about expectations, again the focus needs to be on the actual encounter that looks at empathy, warmth, humanity of the therapist, and understanding even though these may be difficult to define and quantify. However, patient experiences and expectations can be and should be explored in depth but not simply by means of quantitative checklists.

Expectations from a counselling session will differ from those of going to see a nurse in a depot clinic or seeing a physician. Tasman (2002) notes that three psychotherapy processes – empathy, meaning, and doctor-patient relationship – are important in the engagement of patients. Combining these with social or biological interventions may sometimes improve outcomes. The components of empathy, meanings of the experience, and core understanding of the nature of the illness and the person are easy to understand but very difficult to measure and quantify. Negative responses to treatment include increasing demands from the doctors and resolution will then depend upon recognition and gratification of the patient's needs (Gruber & Wood, 1978). It is also quite possible that different therapeutic methods will have different outcomes and these may or may not be influenced by expectations. Nevertheless, expectations will vary. For example, when a patient seeks medical explanations or medical intervention, he or she may very well expect medication and also expect it to work. As evidenced by the placebo effect of medication, the expectations may well be that one particular type of drug or coloured tablet or capsule will work and it does! Similarly, the expectations of therapy from the type of therapist will undoubtedly influence initial engagement. However, its effect on outcome may remain unclear. These findings indicate that different criteria or predictor variables may be needed to evaluate failure (May & Tuma, 1964). It has been shown that patients who seek help for sexual disorders from their doctors believe them to be experts in sexual disorders, which is to be expected (Gorman, 2003).

Three decades ago Moore (1978) emphasized that to be comfortable in the medical environment a psychiatrist had to be comfortable with the skills and values of medicine. These are the core values of professionalism. It is inevitable that some medical symptoms will masquerade as psychiatric disorders, which in turn will exacerbate physical illnesses. Medical training of the psychiatrist therefore influences the patients' expectations that their medical needs will also be looked out for.

It is interesting to note that in an unusual study Sigal et al. (1989) investigated the impact of a nurses' strike on patients functioning on a ward. It was surprising to find that that during the strike patients showed higher responsibility towards ward property and other patients, and there was greater participation in maintaining the ward. Whether this was a reflection of reduced dependence on the staff or whether it was a result of patients asserting some sympathy towards the nurses' cause and therefore were less disruptive is not clear. However, it raises the question of whether the staff infantilize the patients or whether there was a genuine change in the expectations of the patients of the environment and the staff and hence they readjusted. The ratings of behaviour were by the professionals. It would have been useful to have ratings from the relatives and carers.

However, expectations of psychiatrists also include the action of the drugs and response to other physical or medical interventions. Myers and Rosen (1966) noted that psychiatrists did not expect more advances in psychotherapeutic models although drugs, social therapy, and new types of facilities will work better. Thus, expectations of the intervention and environment are also important.

However, in this chapter we emphasize the patients' and other stakeholders' expectations of the psychiatrists as professionals. However, the factors discussed above have to be borne in mind as are a two-way dialogue that does not occur in a vacuum. In an interesting study by Delgado et al. (2007), 360 patients (who had contacted their general practitioners in Spain) were given a 13-item expectation questionnaire. Their expectations for three physical and two psychosocial problems were ascertained. With a response rate of 90%, the authors found that 50% of cases 'with family problems' wanted the doctor alone to make the decision when compared with 68% of patients for 'chest pains'. This may indicate that there are differing expectations according to whether the underlying condition is seen as biomedical or psychosocial. It is also likely that they will expect a doctor to be more interested in physical or medical conditions, hence a different approach. This study indirectly confirms that patient satisfaction and expectation are complex phenomena and are interlinked through a number of mediating factors. Itseih and Kagle (1991) confirmed this hypothesis, noting that the patient's expectations are linked to their socio-demographic factors. In a study from Estonia, Kalda, Polluste, and Lember (2003) found that patients who were not registered with GPs were more likely to have lower levels of expectations from primary care consultation although practice size, patient age, and health status also played a role. Higher levels of satisfaction were associated with physician's understanding (and interestingly punctuality) and effectiveness of prescribed therapy. Giving clear explanations enhanced the possibility of greater satisfaction. The choice of general practitioner and physician is an interesting factor. In health care systems such as the National Health Service in the United Kingdom, the patient's choice of general practitioner and secondary care physician is limited. Thus the satisfaction and expectation will be expected to be low but that is often not the case. It may be that other factors are at play that need to be explored.

Patients expect their doctors to show empathy and in turn doctors too see it as an integral part of their professionalism (Falvo & Smith, 1983; Katic et al., 2001). It is possible to teach medical students as well as trainees about medical professionalism. There are methods that would apply. In a qualitative study Goldie, Bowie, Cotton, and Morrison (2007) found that medical professionalism was considered by tutors and medical students to be related to practitioners' behaviour and experience. Mazor, Clauser, Holtman, and Margolis (2007) found that it is possible to code the doctor–patient interaction using categories that look at the verbal and non-verbal behaviours, how the condition is explored, how the patient is informed, and so on.

Patients also expect their doctors to be efficient, accessible, approachable, honest with them, and not do any harm to them. The reasons doctors are still respected in most settings is that they are seen as being able to provide care at the time of emergency without being greedy or malevolent. The patients and their carers in psychiatric settings expect their clinicians to understand the distress caused by conditions that were often explained as supernatural and difficult to understand and generated stigma. The treatability of certain psychiatric conditions is not always made clear, and often patients and their carers present expecting chronic untreatable conditions. There is thus an implicit expectation that the psychiatrist will hold the patient's hope and contain their anxiety. Doctors are accountable directly to their patients and through them to society. There may be several layers between doctors and society, for example, employer, regulator, and so on.

Carers

Bhugra (2009) reported that in two focus groups with patients and carers in the United Kingdom, common themes emerged. Both groups wanted better information and knowledge about psychiatric conditions than they did before. Access to the Internet may be a positive factor both for carers and patients but the accuracy of information available cannot be verified every time. Thus professionals and professional organizations have a clear obligation to produce and disseminate accurate information as part of their professional duty. Other characteristics of a good psychiatrist identified by the groups were probity and ethics (honesty), being accessible, possessing a good knowledge base, and having excellent communication skills. The psychiatrist as a professional needed to have good interpersonal skills and be a healer. The healer role expected of the psychiatrist raises some interesting issues. Carers' expectations will also influence pathways into care. It is also possible and deserves to be investigated that expectations of the therapeutic encounter will vary according to the need and the time. Emergency assessments carry with them the probability that the crisis needs to be resolved immediately. Those medical students who appear paternalistic in their interviews with patients (and by extension with carers) tend to do worse in their grades in medical school, thereby indicating that there is a change in the way students are assessed. Students who are shy, have poor process skills in gathering information, and hold negative attitudes towards the course perform poorly (Murden, Way, Hudson, & Westman, 2004).

The role of the psychiatrist as a professional as seen by various other stakeholders is important for therapeutic engagement and decrease in stigma.

Psychiatry trainees

With changes in societal and cultural expectations and advances in medical technology, it is inevitable that trainees will respond to these changes and alter the definitions and priorities within the existing definitions of professionalism. In a study by West et al. (2007), over a two-year period, two cohorts of internal medicine trainees in the United States participated in a study of resident competency. Although their medical knowledge over the period increased, empathy decreased, suggesting that the two skills were differently attained. Professionalism requires compassion, integrity, honesty, and respect for patient autonomy. Empathy is a doctor's ability to understand the patient's experience in the context of their being and accordingly convey support and compassion (West et al., 2007). Empathy is the core interaction between the patient and the doctor (Rosenow, 2000). Trainees can be taught professionalism through critical reflective learning (Goldie et al., 2007). Reflective practice is seen as an integral part of professionalism as well as personal development (Gordon, 2003; Kenny, Mann, & Macleod, 2003; Veloshi, Fields, Boex, & Blank, 2005). Professionalism has been assessed in the context of doctor–patient interaction (Mazor et al., 2007). These authors recommend a model where multiple points that cause divergence in ratings can be assessed. The model looks at the encounter as a whole and follows specific behaviours that are evaluated, interpreted, and ratings assigned. Introducing oneself, giving information, explaining, asking questions, and acknowledging patients' concerns are key components of interaction between the doctor and the patient, and these strategies can be taught.

Ratanawongsa et al. (2006) asked 312 residents in three specialties about their attitudes towards professionalism along with what methods were being used to teach them about professionalism. Just over half (169) responded. They were asked to rate 13 principles of professionalism: altruism, respect, sensitivity, accountability, confidentiality, shared decision-making and communication, integrity, duty, competence, managing conflicts of interest, self-awareness, and commitment to excellence and ongoing professional development. The top three barriers to professionalism were time constraints, workload, and patients described as challenging and difficult. Role modelling by faculty and colleagues and culture of the institution were seen as important. In understanding barriers, certainly for psychiatry it is difficult to get away from the notion of difficult or challenging patients. Therefore, this barrier may well differ in psychiatry Time constraints and workload should not necessarily lead to poor professional behaviour. Shared decision-making may be difficult in certain psychiatric conditions when the capacity to make decisions may be lacking or decisions have to be made against the patient's will. Professionalism carries with it remarkable force and deserves full attention, right from medical studentship through to lifelong continuing professional development.

Chard, Eisharkawy, and Newberry (2006) reported on a survey of nearly 24,000 doctors and medical students but with a very low response rate of about 10%. Both trainees and medical students saw medicine as a profession. Clinicians' ethical standards, autonomy, responsibility to the patients and employers were some of the components described as being part of the professionalism. Professionalism related to medicine was also seen as being related to altruism and humility. As the authors point out, medical professionalism is the key to setting standards for patient care, and both training and regulation should be in the purview of the profession.

Adams, O'Reilly, Romm, and James (2006) were able to demonstrate that using Balint groups for training residents in self-assessment was helpful in increasing self-reflection and gaining insight into self and patient care issues. Balint training comprises small groups of clinicians who meet regularly and use the sessions to examine their own experiences and feelings of dealing with patients and learn from each other in the presence of other senior members. Balint groups have also been shown to reduce burnout (Benson & Magraith, 2005). It is self-evident that reflective thinking and discussions will allow the clinicians to be aware of their responses to patients, whether they are difficult or challenging, thereby increasing the levels of professionalism. Unfortunately, in many parts of the world, Balint training is not available. However, it ought to be possible to use other training methods to achieve this.

Public expectations

Increasingly in the United Kingdom, at least, society is becoming risk averse. This means that the homicides caused by patients with mental illness generate banner headlines, not withstanding the fact that the percentage of homicides committed by mentally ill individuals has not changed in the last half century. The advent of community services in the United Kingdom also led to a liberalized view that patients could live and be treated in the community but the general 'not in my backyard' feeling meant that stigma may have actually increased. The public expects the individuals and their families to be safe. The creation of 'the other' allows them to externalize their fears and project them to the other. Equally likely is that they will expect the psychiatrist to contain mentally ill individuals, possibly in an invisible manner. Thus, engaging the public in de-stigmatizing activities goes beyond simple education. Both attitudes and beliefs need to be challenged and changed. The strategy should be that both the psychiatrist and the patients along with their carers work together to provide information and an accurate picture as far as possible. In addition, an open access to the wards will allow the public and stakeholders to see for themselves what treatment strategies and services can achieve and what remains to be done. The public can be and indeed should be engaged in a dialogue to set the standards of health care delivery and the implicit and explicit cost of services that the public may wish to fund. The public is a key stakeholder in identifying needs related to mental illness and their participation will ensure that psychiatrists are able to deliver services which will be emotionally and geographically accessible.

Employers

In health-management organizations and publicly owned health care services, employers have expectations of psychiatrists. They want well-trained professionals who can deliver appropriate services, ensuring that there is a just distribution of finite resources related to the level of need of the patient. Employers expect that the training will be well funded, and yet psychiatrists of the future will be able to work flexibly and deliver services that have clear measurable outcomes. Employers also expect psychiatrists to be advocates for patients, to enable them to gain and maintain employment, quality housing, and at least save social activities. Clear data sets are needed for psychiatric services so that pathways and outcomes can be measured realistically and compared across hospitals and health care services. Psychiatrists are the natural group to help develop these. Furthermore, psychiatrists are natural leaders and should be leading in identifying the psychiatric needs of the local population and then planning, developing, and delivering services that meet those needs. Thus, part of the role of the psychiatrist as a professional is to provide clinical leadership. In settings where service delivery is largely in private hands, the notions of clinical leadership may vary but these would need to be negotiated with local stakeholders. The nature of the relationship between employers and the psychiatrist hinges upon a number of other external factors. Standards for services and training need to be set by the profession itself. However, standards must also be related to the context within which psychiatry is being practised. The relationship of the multidisciplinary team to the employers is markedly complex. The relationship also changes according to specialism.

Caldwelll and Jorm (2000) carried out a postal survey of 673 nurses working in mental health in Australia. The survey included a case vignette either of depression or schizophrenia and asked whether physical (medical), psychological, and lifestyle interventions were helpful, harmful, or neutral. Nurses were more likely than psychiatrists to believe that non-standard interventions such as minerals, vitamins, or naturopathy would help. The surveys with the psychiatrists and the public were carried out at different times. Only 70% of the sample responded. Nurses were more positive than psychiatrists in perceiving herbalists, meditation, relaxation, yoga, counselling, self-help books, hypnosis, special diet, and so on as more helpful for treating schizophrenia.

For depression, the nurses appeared to be more positive about vitamins, herbalists, relaxation, and special diet. Nurses and psychiatrists agreed on many factors in the vignettes. The authors conclude that the nurses' attitudes were a bridge between the public and the psychiatrists, thereby indicating that it may be possible to select interventions that may be helpful and acceptable. Beliefs about illness, its causation, and subsequent treatment will influence expectations. If these findings were upheld in other studies, the beliefs and expectations of nurses of the therapeutic encounter will become more significant as they are able to influence and meet patient expectations.

Whatever the profession, good training is a prerequisite to setting standards and developing reflective thinking. The psychiatrist as a clinical leader can have the vision, which is to do with horizon scanning and preparing for appropriate and relevant response to changing circumstances. Leadership in the clinical sense has also to be seen in the context in which psychiatry is being practised. Clarity and responsibility for vision, collegiality, and holding hope are some of the characteristics of clinical leadership.

Rosen and Dewar (2004) recommend that patient interests should be at the heart of professional practice and the new compact between doctors, government, and the public must be redefined to include other partners such as patient groups and managers. In cases of conflict (which are not rare) there should be a full and frank discussion and the compact must reflect a duty among doctors to engage in improving health services with a reciprocal obligation on the part of the government and mangers to encourage the highest possible professional standards. Rosen and Dewar (2004) argue that medical leadership at an institutional level also needs to be strengthened. The institutional leadership raises interesting notions of who leads – the organization or the individual? The role and responsibility related to leadership and the psychiatrist need to be clarified as a matter of urgency and this volume is a modest attempt in that direction.

Among occupational therapists and social workers, Bhugra (2009) asked questions about the role of professionalism and the role of the psychiatrist. A small number of occupational therapists ($n > 15$) saw the main role of the psychiatrist as that of a diagnostician and leader, although some felt that diagnoses change over time. The main qualities of the psychiatrist were related to listening and communicating. They support the team and can direct the culture and philosophy of the team. Other skills expected of a good psychiatrist include teaching, educating, and evaluating evidence. Being clear about expectations and being taken seriously were seen as part of the professionalism.

A small group of social workers ($n = 35$) also responded to a web-based questionnaire. Their responses also suggested that psychiatrists needed to be team players, patient focused, good listeners, empathic, holistic in approach, reflective and reflexive, good communicators, compassionate, and giving priority to the patient's needs.

Although both the professional groups have small numbers and may not be entirely representative of the professions, there occur common themes of being a team player, a good communicator, patient-focused, a good listener, and empathic. Patients and their carers and the psychiatrists all think the same way, and their expectations of the psychiatrists are the same as those of psychiatric trainees and psychiatrists themselves, thereby indicating that it is possible to identify common skills, competencies, and attitudes. It also confirms that all the key stakeholders working in the field who were approached have similar views of professionalism in the twenty-first century. Exploratory work with nurses and psychologists is currently under way.

In the latter half of the twentieth century, the values of professionalism relate to medicine in general and psychiatry in particular in the United Kingdom at least were under serious threat. The profession needs to take charge and redefine the constituents of professionalism with key stakeholders and then incorporate these into training psychiatrists of the future.

Conclusion

There is little doubt that professionalism in psychiatry is extremely important and it is up to the profession to explore this with stakeholders. Some stakeholders may hold differing views, but it should be possible to explore common strands across different disciplines. Psychiatry has an obligation as a science to be evidence-based and apply the evidence appropriately. However, as an art psychiatry has to engage patients, their carers, and not only other members of the team, but on their behalf psychiatry has to speak to society at large and get their agreement through their representatives. Diagnosis and managing medication are one aspect of the professional role which psychiatrists play, but medical management will include much more than medication. That is the challenge for psychiatry – to define it and act on it to deliver holistic and appropriate services that will be used by the patients and the carers, who will then have full confidence in the profession.

References

Adams, K. E., O'Reilly, M., Romm, J., & James, K. (2006). Effects of Balint training on resident professionalism. *American Journal of Obstetrics and Gynecology,* **195**, 1431–1437.

Benson, J., & Magraith, K. (2005). Compassion fatigue and burnout: The role of Balint groups. *Australian Family Physician,* **34**, 497–498.

Bhugra, D. (2009). Professionalism and psychiatry: Past, present, future. *Australasian Psychiatry, 17*, 357–359.

Chard, D., Eisharkawy, A., & Newberry, N. (2006). Medical professionalism: the trainees' views. *Clinical Medicine, 6*, 68–71.

Delgado, A., Lopez-Fernandez, L. A., Dias Luna, J., Gill, N., Jimenez, M., & Puga, A. (2007). Patient expectations are not always the same. *Journal of Epidemiology and Community Health, 62*, 427–434.

Falvo, D. R., & Smith, J. K. (1983). Assessing residents' behavioural science skills: Patients' views of physician patient interaction. *The Journal of Family Practice, 17*, 479–483.

Goldie, J., Bowie, A., Cotton, P., & Morrison, J. (2007). Teaching professionalism in the early years of a medical curriculum: A qualitative study. *Medical Education, 41*, 610–617.

Gordon, J. (2003). Fostering students' personal and professional development in medicine: A new framework for PPD. *Medical Education, 37*, 341–349.

Gorman, J. M. (2003). Filling in the gaps and making the connections: Sexual disorders in neuroscience. *CNS Spectrums, 8*, 170.

Gruber, L. N., & Wood, A. M. (1978). Negative treatment responses in psychiatry. *Journal of Clinical Psychiatry, 39*, 279–283.

Kalda, R., Polluste, K., & Lember, M. (2003). Patient satisfaction with care is associated with personal choice of physician. *Health Policy, 64*, 55–62.

Katic, M., Budak, A., Ivankovic, D., et al. (2001). Patients' views on the professional behaviour of family physicians. *Family Practice, 18*, 42–47.

Kenny, N., Mann, K., & Macleod, H. (2003). Role modelling in physicians' professional formation: Reconsidering an essential but untapped educational strategy. *Academic Medicine, 78*, 1203–1210.

May, P. R. A., & Tuma, A. H. (1964). Choice of criteria for the assessment of treatment outcome. *Journal of Psychiatric Research, 2*, 199–209.

Mazor, K. M., Clauser, B. E., Holtman, M., & Margolis, M. J. (2007). Evaluation of missing data in an assessment of professional behaviors. *Academic Medicine, 82*, S44–S47.

Moore, G. L. (1978). The adult psychiatrist in the medical environment. *The American Journal of Psychiatry, 135*, 413–419.

Murden, R. A., Way, D. P., Hudson, A., & Westman, J. A. (2004). Professionalism deficiencies in a first quarter doctor–patient relationship course predict poor clinical performance in medical school. *Academic Medicine, 79*, 546–548.

Myers, J. M., & Rosen, H. B. (1966). Psychiatrists' current attitudes about psychiatric treatment. *Comprehensive Psychiatry, 7*, 232–239.

Ratanawongsa, N., Bolen, S., Howell, E. E., et al. (2006). Residents' perceptions of professionalism in training and practice: Barriers, promoters and duty hour requirements. *Journal of General Internal Medicine, 21*, 758–763.

Rosen, R. A., & Dewar, S. (2004). *On Being a Doctor: Redefining Medical Professionalism for Better Patient Care.* London: King's Fund.

Rosenow, E. C., (2000). Recertifying in the art of medicine: What I would tell the young physicians. *Mayo Clinic Proceedings, 75*, 865–868.

Sigal, M., Diamont, J., Bacalu, A., et al. (1989). The effects of a nurses' strike on the functioning of chronic patients. *Hospital & Community Psychiatry, 40*, 409–411.

Tasman, A. (2002). Lost in the DSM-IV: Empathy, meaning and the doctor–patient relationship. *Academic Psychiatry,* **26**, 38–44.

Veloshi, J., Fields, S. K., Boex, J. R., & Blank, L. L. (2005). Measuring professionalism: a review of studies with instruments reported in the literature between 1962 and 2002. *Academic Medicine,* **80**, 366–370.

West, C. P., Huntington, J. L. Huschka, M. M., et al. (2007). A prospective study of the relationship between medical knowledge and professionalism among internal medicine residents. *Academic Medicine,* **82**, 587–592.

Chapter 7

Training and professionalism

Greg Lydall and Amit Malik

Introduction

Who, in future, will be providing professional medical expertise when we, our child, or our parent develops mental illness? What kinds of psychiatrists, with what values and skills, are we training, and should we be training? The qualities defining a professional have been explored elsewhere in this book. The psychiatric trainees' perspective on professionalism and society encompasses those years of training during which a general medical graduate becomes a specialist physician of the mind. During this period, the trainee must undergo a process of 'systematic required training' to a gain a breadth and depth of 'technical specialized knowledge' towards a service-oriented ethical code found in professionals (Starr, 1982). He or she must develop a working understanding of the complex interplay of mind, brain, and body; of the branches of psychiatry; and of the health and social service and its governance. Trainees must further acquire clinical and non-clinical skills, experience, expertise, and confidence in practicing in the specialty which, above all others deals in the uncertainties of the human experience. Bhugra (2008) suggests that 'psychiatrists are, arguably, best placed to deal with ambiguity and uncertainty and we need to enhance these skills. Reflective practice and emotional intelligence are important parts of self-awareness and growth which we need to encourage.' Finally, the trainee must internalize the character, rights, and responsibilities relevant to both sides of psychiatry's implicit contract with society (Bhugra, 2008).

This contract is set within an evolving society. Of particular relevance to psychiatric training are changes in the following:

- models of care (increasingly community-based care),
- postgraduate training models (from an apprenticeship model to competency-based curricula; from a medical firm to a shift system),
- national health policy and working hours (varying by nation),
- mental health legislation (the tension between personal freedoms and risk aversion),

- attitudes towards psychiatry both within the professions and the public (generally improving but from a low baseline),
- patient knowledge and expectations (increasing, as is litigation),
- health and wider economies (cost management and a shift towards outcomes-linked funding during a period of relative economic austerity),
- professional culture (external management and regulation of professionals).

This chapter will cover the main training challenges of relevance to psychiatric trainees within this context, highlight current ambiguities, and search for solutions.

Models of care

Probably the largest shift in psychiatric models of care has been from long-term institutional care towards care in the community. There is increasing evidence of the therapeutic and economic value of community- and home-based treatment for mental illnesses that previously would have been treated in hospital (Marshall & Lockwood 1998; Wright, Catty, Watt, & Burns, 2004). Both patients and trainees thus spend far less time in hospital, which for most patients is undeniably an improvement. For trainees however, this risks less-concentrated clinical hospital exposure owing to the less-intense and structured nature of community services. Yet a small but significant percentage of people with mental illness will at some point benefit from in-hospital treatment (owing to risks to self or others, failure of community treatment, poor engagement, diagnostic uncertainty, illness, or other factors). Psychiatrists will thus need to retain inpatient skills in addition to learning community-based treatment. Psychiatric services are thus likely to require psychiatric expertise in various forms of community treatment (home treatment teams, assertive outreach teams, early intervention services) (Department of Health, 1998) and hospital treatment (open, locked, intensive care, and rehabilitation wards.)

To mitigate against poor recruitment and burnout among UK consultant psychiatrists, a model of care entitled New Ways of Working (NWW) was developed by the Department of Health in collaboration with the Royal College of Psychiatrists and other groups (Department of Health, 2005). The NWW aimed to empower multidisciplinary team members in managing psychiatric cases, leaving the most complex cases and medication issues to psychiatrists. Implementation of diverse interpretations of the NWW model has resulted in a wide variation in service quality.

Critics of the NWW system suggest that it has been used as a cost-saving measure to employ fewer doctors – non-medical workers display a wide variation in skill levels – leading to cases of inappropriate or frankly unsafe treatment and ironically to further isolation of consultant psychiatrists.

Non-medical prescribing, while allowing for enhanced skills and roles, has shifted the emphasis further away from medical responsibility. Although it takes 5 to 6 years to train a doctor to prescribe without supervision, nurses and pharmacists are increasingly regulated to prescribe, with significantly less pharmacology training, albeit in limited areas. Detractors of both non-medical assessments and prescribing note that referrers from UK primary care to specialist psychiatric services can no longer expect their patients to be assessed by a doctor (Craddock et al., 2008). Senior members of the profession have raised concerns about the impact on patient safety and care, loss of the medical model, and unintended negative consequences including those on training (Craddock et al., 2008; St John-Smith, 2009). Little has been published on specific training consequences of an altered training milieu.

Impacts on training may include that trainees may now see fewer yet more complex patients, with a narrower range of psychopathology and prescribing under the above models. It must be remembered that all these factors occur in the context of reduced hours and shift working (discussed below.) To differentiate and manage complex cases as consultants, trainees will need to build on initial experience with routine cases. Consultants as trainers will need to see and supervise trainees with routine cases and prescribing, gradually increasing in complexity as trainee competence improves. Thus if training remains embedded within consultant roles, consultants will need to see both simple and complex cases in the time available for training.

Working hours

Mastering the skills of a psychiatrist requires adequate clinical exposure to training appropriate tasks over sufficient time. Hours of working (and thus hours available for training) have decreased steadily in the majority of specialties in Europe, the United Kingdom (Cairns, Hendry, Leather, & Moxham, 2008), and the United States (Philbert, 2002). In many countries doctors in training were expected to work 100 or more hours per week until recently. In Europe hours worked have been reduced step-wise by legislation to the current 48 hours. US residents' hours have been reduced after considerable debate within the Academies, although not to the same degree as in Europe. Craft specialties like surgery in particular have expressed grave concerns that the reduction in hours will lead to reductions in training experience. However because in the United Kingdom training posts are funded separately from service posts, several organizations argue that training must take precedence over service in the remaining hours (British Medical Association, 2009) The blurred boundaries (and indeed overlap) between 'training' and 'service' have not helped the debate move on. The British Medical Association and NHS have agreed that junior doctors should maximize their training in the hours available by focusing on training appropriate tasks; inappropriate work is considered better done by other staff groups. This leads to potential tensions over complicated definitions of 'appropriate' work and diffusion of responsibility. It also risks undermining the tradition (and indeed societal expectation) that medical professionals will do whatever needs to be done in healing their patient, whether it is good for their training or not.

Another implication of a shorter shift system is the requirement for safe handover, which often does not translate well in psychiatry. There is no production line that can be stopped; professional duty of care does not end with the shift. Continuity of care is valued by both professionals and patients, and arguably allows for increased efficiency because less duplication of effort (history taking, investigations, and handover) is required. Furthermore, continuity is important in training: rapid feedback on diagnostic accuracy and soundness of management plans as well as the experience of walking with a patient from illness to recovery are essential to training psychiatric experts. An area of tension between trainees and hospital managers has been the requirement to 'drop tools' to work within hours limits, yet no professional psychiatrist would abandon a patient mid-sentence to meet working hours demands. More discrete work periods require robust handover arrangements for safety. Handover is a skill that requires training, assessment, and quality control through clinical governance.

Psychiatric emergency and out-of-hours experience are a vital part of specialist training in psychiatry. Out-of-hours work allows for experience of different pathologies more likely to appear at night (notably delirium, self-harm, substance misuse, psychosis) with less senior availability, wherein clinical decision-making, team working, and judgement skills are refined. Partly to reduce doctor-hours worked, non-medical psychiatric liaison teams – often staffed by experienced senior nurses – have increased. Although this has in many cases improved availability and responsiveness of mental health services, there are two major drawbacks. The first is that the most acute and complex cases presenting emergently are thus increasingly not being seen by a medical professional. Second there is a real risk that junior trainees may simply not see enough clinical cases to gain sufficient competence, with clear implications for treatment and training. In the United Kingdom this essential experience continues to be eroded, despite guidance from the Royal College (Royal College of Psychiatrists, 2008) If psychiatrists of the future are to develop and maintain their emergency psychiatry skills, and provide the comprehensive, safe service expected by society, then such training should remain an integral part of any training programme.

Training reforms

Traditionally, training models have required a minimum time served and an exit trial or examination whereby skills are proven to the satisfaction of senior professionals. This has been termed the apprenticeship model. Newer competence-based models require sequential assessment and proof of specific competencies with less emphasis on time in training. A further major shift has been from a medical hierarchy to a multidisciplinary team-based model. A societal and political desire to regulate risk by standardizing and quantifying exactly what skills doctors learn in training arose. In the United Kingdom, specialization standards were set and enforced by professional bodies usually medical Royal Colleges.

Over time, the colleges were perceived as self-serving and independent-minded, and a new quasi-non-governmental body was promulgated to oversee all postgraduate medical training (Department of Health, 2003) Detailed curricula have been developed in various countries such that trainees' competencies can be assessed against a standard. Examples include the UK's Royal College of Psychiatrists (College, 2008) and the Canadian Medical Education Directives for Specialists (CanMEDS) curriculum (Canada, 1996). Concerns were raised about the tools used to assess clinical competence, particularly with questions as to their validity and reliability (Mickelson & MacNeily, 2008). The reduction in hours worked (see above) and the growth of shift systems have interrupted the apprentice/team training experience. On the positive side these developments may mean exposure to a variety of trainers and disciplines and more explicit criteria defining a 'fit for purpose' specialist psychiatrist. On the negative side, first the continuity of training and patient care so long a part of medicine have been disturbed. Second, the tools for assessing competencies, at least in the United Kingdom, are still being developed and refined. It is thus important to maintain some minimum criteria as evidence of standards. Both time and experience may be considered until there is greater confidence in the delivery and assessment of a competence-based model.

The UK postgraduate training system has undergone two major reforms in a decade-and-a-half: The Calman reforms (Calman, 1993) and modernizing medical careers (MMC; Donaldson, 2002). The United States and other countries have undergone their own reorganizations. The UK changes were intended to remove bottlenecks between upwards training grades and improve the flexibility and efficiency of the training systems. The most recent UK reform, MMC, was implemented in 2007 across England, Scotland, Wales, and Northern Ireland with regrettable consequences. With no significant expansion in training numbers, and despite warnings, the new system resulted in 32,000 doctors applying (or reapplying in many cases) for about 22,000 posts

UK-wide through a defective electronic application system and an overstretched selection system. The consequences included significant service and career disruption, trainee distress, and career disillusionment (Lydall, Malik, Blizard, & Bhugra, 2009). There was also a loss of faith in the postgraduate training system and the professional bodies responsible for maintaining standards and protecting the profession. The process and effects were the subject of an independent review that made numerous far-reaching recommendations (Tooke, 2007). The Tooke report interestingly also compares postgraduate training systems in several countries for the interested reader. A series of unintended consequences of MMC include less flexibility (owing to a fixed run-through programme allowing little time out), earlier specialty pathway choice (owing to pressure to enter training, and a lack of stand-alone 'taster' jobs), and a delayed dissatisfaction effect (trainees forced to select second-choice specialties during the MMC debacle just to ensure employment or geographic stability).

In UK psychiatry, a further subtle shift occurred towards service and away from training during the most recent training reform. Previously, advanced trainees in psychiatry were both supernumerary and entitled to a day's research training and a day's clinical special interest training. This was protected by the Royal College to allow attainment of educationally agreed skills, which would not normally be accessible in a standard training post. Despite published evidence of the worth of this protected time in moulding the varied skills of the higher specialist trainee, there was a perception among senior doctors and medical managers that use of this time was inefficient at best, and detracting from the core service at worst. The amount of protected training and research time was halved in the MMC reform with College agreement. This decision effectively handed employing organizations an extra day a week of senior medical expertise, with no apparent plan as to what training would be received in its place. Trainees perceived this as a loss of equitability, flexibility, competitiveness, and opportunity (Lydall & Bourke, 2009). The loss of protected research time leaves little opportunity for non-academic trainees to fulfil their professional obligations to participate in research as required in the General Medical Council's 'Good doctor' framework (GMC, 2005). Loss of protected clinical special interest sessions requires an alternative method of developing sub-speciality interests which both employers and society will value.

Policymakers are increasingly emphasizing the importance of developing defined management and leadership skills in medical specialists. Two influential UK documents, the Darzi report (Health, 2008) and the Medical Leadership Competency Framework (MLCF; Colleges, 2009) highlight these requirements. What has not been made clear is, given the reduced time available for training and increased knowledge and specialization, how much time to allocate to management and leadership training. Perhaps more crucial is robust training in the difficult ethical conflicts occurring when medical managers must choose between balancing budgets and cutting services.

Academic training

In the United Kingdom, mental health research receives only 6.5% of funding compared with 15% for neurology, and 25% for cancer (Royal College of Psychiatrists, 2007) This low level persists despite the high prevalence and chronicity of some mental illness. Academic psychiatry is thought to be in a crisis in many countries (Kupfer, et al., 2009). In addition, much psychopharmacology research is industry-led leading to potential conflicts of interest and giving further ammunition to the anti-psychiatry lobby (Rothman, et al., 2009). Recent efforts to address this funding shortfall include academic tracks within clinical training and ring-fenced research funding, particularly in the United States with the National Institutes for Health (NIH), and in the United Kingdom with the National Institute for Health Research (NIHR) and Medical Research Council (MRC). These transfusions, although welcome and important, may be insufficient given the chronic anaemia of research investment. In addition, time available for research during training is decreasing (see above) with increasing service pressures, yet new training models require explicit and quantifiable research outcomes. With fewer academic posts available, and less research emphasis in psychiatry, we risk losing our analytical and academic trainees to other specialities. Psychiatry is grossly under-researched. It seems prudent to invest in improved understanding and treatment in the short term that will actually reduce service requirements in the long term. What psychiatry and its patients thus need is time and resource for independent academic-led research to shine light into the darkness of our understanding. With increased resources and public appetite, the specialty will make good progress towards reducing morbidity and mortality associated with mental illness. With improved understanding of the biological and social underpinnings of psychiatric illness, innovative and safe treatments may be developed to the benefit of a society currently burdened with mental illness.

Funding

Psychiatric care receives 10% of the UK and 6% of the US health budgets, respectively (WHO, 2008). The underfunding of mental health services relative to the prevalence, chronicity, and disability associated with mental illness affects not just on public health but also on services, training, and recruitment.

Even in countries with higher levels of socialized health, psychiatric services and training budgets are often relatively under-resourced and overstretched. This has various knock-on effects including increased strain on the service and its workers, an unsatisfactory patient experience, and presenting an unattractive impression to medical students. Various professional bodies have raised the issue of chronic underfunding with the Royal College of Psychiatrists' Fair Deal programme highlighting the need for **F**unding; **A**ccess to services; **I**n-patient services; **R**ecovery and rehabilitation; **D**iscrimination and stigma; **E**ngagement with service users and carers; **A**vailability of psychological therapies; **L**inking physical and mental health (College, 2008). Future service funding approaches are increasingly likely to be linked to case turnover, quality outcomes, and 'customer satisfaction'. These approaches have unique challenges in psychiatry where quality improvements are often not clear-cut or easy to measure, and 'customers' may at times be required by society to be treated against their will. If implemented thoughtlessly, such funding reforms risk worsening an already dire funding situation (Fairbairn, 2007).

Imminent changes in funding of postgraduate training budgets in the context of underfunded facilities in which training is delivered creates further strain on the training system. In the United Kingdom, ring-fencing of training budgets is being considered to protect training funds from diversion towards supporting services. Because of the blurred boundaries and overlap between service and training, this approach risks making the monetary value of hosting trainees more explicit. Where organizations consider trainees poor value for money, the range of training opportunities may actually decrease. Anecdotal evidence suggests that recent alterations in training funding streams may actually have destabilized the finances of some NHS training institutions.

Recruitment challenges and shortage of specialists

Society deserves high-quality doctors choosing psychiatry. Medical students and young doctors considering a career in psychiatry are rarer and perhaps braver than those considering other pathways. Attitudes towards psychiatry are positive upon starting medical school but decline during medical school towards graduation (Goldacre, Turner, Fazel, & Lambert 2005).There is an acknowledged chronic worldwide shortage of psychiatrists and other mental health workers in the context of chronic underfunding of services (WHO, 2008). The putative causes are multiple and have been reviewed by Thomas and Thomas (2008). Our understanding of the complex area of career choice is limited by methodological considerations in that we can only infer a causal relationship from the current literature. To encourage more high-quality doctors to choose psychiatry will require changes at several levels. In Table 7.1

Table 7.1 Suggested strategies to improve recruitment and retention into psychiatry (adapted from Seed, Lydall et al., in press)

Select the right sort of people into medical school who might become psychiatrists, that is, those with arts and social sciences qualifications, some experience of a family member with a mental illness, and positive attitudes towards mental illness (Brockington & Mumford, 2002); urban backgrounds, with low scores on tests of authoritarianism, high tolerance of uncertainty and liberal political views (Eagle & Marcos 1980); female gender and overall goals in life (Buddeberg-Fischer, Klaghofer et al. 2006)
Positive medical school experiences such as psychology and sociology modules, sufficient length of clinical placement exposure, setting of clinical placement with sufficient exposure to motivated patients and effective forms of treatment, availability of special study modules and electives (Manassis, Katz, Lofchy, & Wiesenthal, S2006; Mihalynuk, Leung, Fraser, Bates, & Snadden, . 2006); High-quality teaching and availability of good role models (Shelley & Webb, 1986; McParland, Noble, Livingston, McManus, 2003; Maidment, Livingston, Katona, McParland, & Noble, 2004; Kuhnigk, Strebel, Schilauske, & Jueptner, 2007) and addressing negative attitudes from other specialities (Creed & Goldberg,1987)
Positive postgraduate factors such as availability of early clinical posts in psychiatry, work-life balance, remuneration (Goldacre, Turner, Fazel, & Lambert 2005; Lambert, Turner, Fazel, & Goldacre, 2006; Thomas & Thomas 2008; Wigney, Parker et al. 2007)
Improve public awareness of the positive roles of psychiatrists and address public and professional stigma towards mental illness and those who diagnose and treat it.

we suggest policy and personal changes that will project psychiatry as the exciting, rewarding, creative, and integrative specialty that it is.

Professional bodies and 'deprofessionalization'

Another concerning development is the repeated attempts by UK health employers to devalue the end point of specialty training. The quality and affordability of consultants has been directly questioned by NHS Employers, one of the largest employers in the world (NHS Employers, 2008). Here the employers suggest that reduced clinical 'engagement' by consultants in some specialities reduce their value for money, that future consultants may be undertrained, that 'differential roles' for specialists may be appropriate, and that patients are less concerned with being treated by a doctor than with having 'experienced, qualified people' treating them. The differential roles would be seen as cost saving and have been referred to as a 'sub-consultant grade' that has been repeatedly rejected by the British Medical Association, the professional body representing doctors in the United Kingdom. Despite significant expansion in consultant numbers the United Kingdom is still arguably under-doctored, and the NHS is underfunded as a proportion of gross domestic product compared to European levels. The NHS employers have publically stated that not all doctors who hold a certificate of completion of (specialist) training (CCT) will be able to work in consultant posts. The remainder would move into non-training posts that are primarily geared towards service provision (Newshound, 2009). The latter inevitably divides doctors into those on two pathways, with one cohort headed towards an inferior training standard. These 'sub-consultants' are likely to be paid less (NHS employers have stated that the NHS cannot afford more consultants), with fewer opportunities for career progression. This outcome stands in stark contrast to what any patient deserves, especially the mentally ill: assessment and treatment by a highly trained consultant.

Updating mental health legislation in England and Wales to reflect changes in mental health treatment was accompanied by several other significant amendments. These included elimination of the psychiatrist's exclusivity as legally responsible medical officers (responsible for the treatment of detained patients) (Mental Health Act, 2007). In new legislation, any 'clinician' meeting minimum qualifications (including first level nurses and psychologists) and experience may complete a two-day course and become a 'responsible clinician'. Thus in theory decisions about ongoing detention, ward leave, treatment, and also discharge from detention no longer require a medical doctor with years of comprehensive undergraduate and postgraduate training. For now however, medication decisions require consultation with a medical practitioner. Given the current direction of travel away from medical leadership and responsibility, future legislation may conceivably not require any medical input. Senior psychiatrists have questioned whether psychiatrists were subject to a 'deprofessionalization agenda' (Brown & Bhugra, 2007). This is because their traditional roles were seen to be eroded by reforms like NWW, non-medical prescribing, and non-medical roles in mental health legislation.

This conflict highlights the tension between time and opportunity available for training and society's skills requirements. It is unclear whether increasing specialization or maintenance of broad-based skills is the optimum way forward (Anonymous, 1994; Goodwin & Geddes, 2007). Balancing sufficient clinical exposure during training to reach a level of clinical expertise with the needs of the service requires ongoing energies. When service needs impinge on training, professional bodies will be best placed to protect training. Professional bodies specific to psychiatry include medical royal colleges (in the United Kingdom, the Royal College of Psychiatrists), the American Psychiatric Association, and the European Psychiatric Association. In broader medical terms, the British and American Medical Associations have multiple roles including trade union, negotiation, scientific policy, and education and training roles. Professional organizations often have public influence and political lobbying power. It is essential that professional bodies uphold 'the well-being of others above the professional's personal gain,' (Racy, 1990) When service requirements change, and standards are threatened by short-term political goals, these same bodies should lead in defining training curricula and standards, professional culture, and the higher ideals characteristic of such bodies.

Know and heal thyself

The phrase, 'physician heal thyself' has several interpretations of relevance to professionalism. The most obvious is perhaps where doctors self-diagnose and self-treat. It also refers to the expectation that doctors are somehow super-human and less vulnerable to human foibles and illnesses. Finally, the phrase hints at a higher level of self-knowledge perhaps imparted through years of specialized training.

Physicians are reported to have high levels of stress, mental illness, and substance misuse problems as well as higher suicide rates (Firth-Cozens, 1999; Hawton, Clements, Sakarovitch, Simkin, & Deeks, 2001).

Self-regulation as a crucial component of professionalism implies the need for systematic reliable recognition of health and performance problems. Detection by others is one side of the coin. Self-awareness and thus self-recognition by individual professionals is the other. Awareness alone is insufficient – knowledge of appropriate and required actions, once a problem is detected, is essential.

Recognition of one's own level of functioning, and possible impairment, along with appropriate help-seeking are required in the annual UK physician appraisal that is soon to be regulated by the GMC. The focus needs to move towards preparation for the strains of professional practice, both in the training process and as practicing specialists.

It is felt that self-regulation may improve through better training in personal health and performance management within the professions. This training might intuitively occur during undergraduate education and be reinforced throughout specialization and beyond. Against the argument is the lack of evidence of efficacy of such an approach. Good practice examples of such training include Resident Wellness Programmes (e.g., at the University of Toronto, Canada: www.pgme.utoronto.ca/wellness.) This programme covers proactive educational and self-awareness modules, and a pastoral support and referral system.

Should psychiatry trainees be required to receive personal therapy? This policy area has arguments for and against. Less than 2% of US residency programmes require psychotherapy; in the United States and United Kingdom it is typically mandatory only in psychoanalytic sub-specialty training. Under half of US training programmes recommended personal psychotherapy (Daly, 1998) and the UK guidance is notably silent on the issue. Take-up of personal therapy may be decreasing (Haak & Kaye, 2009). Personal therapy has been found beneficial for psychiatry residents with emotional and personal difficulties (Wallace & Tisdall, 1991). Advantages of mandatory therapy are improved insight, responsiveness and sensitivity, and mental health. Disadvantages are cost, time, lack of evidence of efficacy, and cost-effectiveness, and an increasingly biological emphasis in psychiatry. Barriers include cost, training demands, and possibly intra-professional stigma. This is an area for further debate and policy direction from within the profession. Currently we suggest a minimum of an integrated trainee wellness module into training. Useful themes (derived from programmes above) are listed on Table 7.2.

We conclude that a healthy self-knowledge as part of a proactive approach towards wellness during training, and continued within post-specialization development is increasingly important. Improved preparation for the complexities of the psychiatrist's role is likely to advance personal aspects of self-regulation and thus benefit both practitioners and patients.

Conclusion

There are many challenges ahead to ensure that professional healers of the mind continue to build public trust so that they may practice their art for the betterment of society. It seems that society and doctors cherish the role of healer and professional. Increasing awareness of the challenges in training psychiatrists of the future and open discussion about their roles are positive developments. Calls for explicit teaching of professional values (Cruess & Cruess, 1997), and physician self-awareness modules are further signs of progress.

Table 7.2 Suggested themes for a trainee wellness programme

- Epidemiology of physical and mental health problems among doctors
- Self awareness (personality, strengths, vulnerabilities)
- Stress management
- Optimizing lifestyle factors
- Personal therapy: the evidence for and against
- Basic cognitive behavioural principles for self-application
- Early warning signs of possible problems
- Local and national sources of help
- Detecting and managing colleagues in distress
- Regulatory attitudes towards impaired doctors

Table 7.3 Professionalism and training: Priority policy and research questions

1. Training
   - Debate and direction on specialization or generalization (in time available for training)
   - Debate and direction on medical management (ethical dilemmas and skill level required in postgraduate training of limited time)
   - Debate and direction on role of personal psychotherapy
   - Training in public education role
   - Resurrect physical medicine skills
   - Strengthen physical medical skills

2. Aetiology and treatment
   - Research in basic sciences, early/formative years, and translational ('from bench to bedside')
   - Investment in novel physical and psychological treatments
   - Increase the evidence base for applicability and efficacy of psychotherapeutic techniques and contingency management

3. Policy
   - Professional bodies actively educate public, professions (including our own) and commissioners/purchasers of services on crucial role of broad psychiatric assessment and treatment
   - Debate and direction on boundaries of psychiatric illness, that is, requiring psychiatric as opposed to non-specific psychosocial assessment and treatment
   - Active recruitment to psychiatry program to nurture and select the best doctors into the profession
   - Robust workforce planning to provide clearer pathways and employment opportunity data

4. Personal responsibility
   - Increasing public education of modifiable lifestyle factors in mental illness
   - Debate and direction on explicit contract of patient personal responsibility (including concordance with treatment, lifestyle modification, and consequences of contract breaking)

Yet there are ongoing reforms to training these healers that may disadvantage society in future. There is a concern that, for the sake of political expediency, an unrealistic desire for risk management, and short-term cost savings, that society may be mortgaging the present to secure the future. In Table 7.3 we set out a list of priority questions for debate and research within and without the profession. It is hoped that engagement in these crucial areas will enhance the direction and content of training programmes for psychiatrists of the future.

References

Anonymous. (1994). Molecules and minds. *Lancet*, **343**, 681–682.

Bhugra, D. (2008). Renewing psychiatry's contract with society. *Psychiatric Bulletin*, **32**, 281–283.

British Medical Association. (2009). EWTD briefing paper from the Junior Doctors Committee: Facing the challenges of the EWTD. Retrieved from 30 June 2010 http://www.bma.org.uk/employmentandcontracts/working_arrangements/hours/euroworktim.jsp

Brockington, I., & Mumford, D. B. (2002). Recruitment into psychiatry [see comment]. *British Journal of Psychiatry,* **180,** 307–312.

Buddeberg-Fischer, B., Klaghofer, R. Abel, T., & Buddeberg, C. (2006). Swiss residents speciality choices – impact of gender, personality traits, career motivation and life goals. *BMC Health Services Research,* **6,** 137.

Cairns, H., Hendry, B., Leather, A., & Moxham, J . (2008). Outcomes of the European working time directive. *BMJ,* **337,** a942.

Calman, K. (1993). *Hospital Doctors: Training for the Future. The Report of the Working Group on Specialist Medical Training.* London: Department of Health.

Canada, R. C. o. P. a. S. o. (1996) CanMEDs Framework.

Craddock, N., Antebi, D., Attenburrow, M-J, et al. (2008). Wake-up call for British psychiatry. *The British Journal of Psychiatry,* **193,** 6–9.

Creed, F., & Goldberg, D. (1987). Doctors' interest in psychiatry as a career. *Medical Education,* **21,** 235–243.

Cruess, R. L., & Cruess, S. R. (1997). Teaching medicine as a profession in the service of healing. *Academic Medicine,* **72,** 941–952.

Daly, K. A. (1998). Attitudes of U.S. psychiatry residencies about personal psychotherapy for psychiatry residents. *Academic Psychiatry,* **22,** 223–228.

Department of Health. (2003). *The General and Specialist Medical Practice (Education, Training and Qualifications) Order.* London: Author.

Department of Health. (2005). *New Ways of Working for Psychiatrists: Enhancing Effective, Person-Centred Services through New Ways of Working in Multidisciplinary and Multiagency Contexts. Final Report but Not the eND of the Story.* London: Author.

Donaldson, L. (2002). *Unfinished Business-Proposals for Reform of the Senior House Officer Grade.* C. M. O. f. London: Department of Health.

Eagle, P. F., & Marcos, L. R. (1980). Factors in medical students choice of psychiatry. *American Journal of Psychiatry,* **137,** 423–427.

Fairbairn, A. (2007). Payment by results in mental health: the current state of play in England. *Advances in Psychiatric Treatmen,* **13,** 3–6.

Firth-Cozens, J. (1999). *The Psychological Problems of Doctors. In Stress in Health Professionals: Psychological and Organizational Causes and Interventions.* Chichester: John Wiley & Sons.

Goldacre, M. J., Turner, G., Fazel, S., & Lambert, T. (2005). Career choices for psychiatry: national surveys of graduates of 1974-2000 from UK medical schools. *The British Journal of Psychiatry,* **186,** 158–164.

Goldacre, M. J., Turner, G., Fazel, S., & Lambert, T. (2005). Career choices for psychiatry: national surveys of graduates of 1974–2000 from UK medical schools. [erratum appears in Br J Psychiatry. 2005 **186,** 357]. *British Journal of Psychiatry,* **186,** 158–164.

Goodwin, G., & Geddes, J. (2007). What is the heartland of psychiatry? *British Journal of Psychiatry,* **191,** 189–191.

Haak, J. L., & Kaye, D.(2009). Personal psychotherapy during residency training: A survey of psychiatric residents. *Academic Psychiatry,* **33,** 323–326.

Hawton, K., Clements, A., Sakarovitch, C., Simkin, S., & Deeks, J. (2001). Suicide in doctors. *Journal of Epidemiology and Community Health,* **55**, 296–300.

Kuhnigk, O., Strebel, B., Schilauske, J., & Jueptner, M. (2007). Attitudes of medical students towards psychiatry: effects of training, courses in psychiatry, psychiatric experience and gender. *Advances in Health Sciences Education,* **12**, 87–101.

Kupfer, D. J., Schatzberg, A. F., Grochocinski, V. J., Dunn, L. O., Kelley, K. A., & O'Hara, R. A. (2009). The Career Development Institute for Psychiatry: An innovative, longitudinal program for physician-scientists. *Academic Psychiatry,* **33**, 313–318.

Lambert, T. W., Turner, G., Fazel, S., & Goldacre, M. J. (2006). Reasons why some UK medical graduates who initially choose psychiatry do not pursue it as a long-term career. *Psychological Medicine,* **36**, 679–684.

Lydall, G., Malik, A., Blizard, R., & Bhugra, D. (2009). Psychological impact of systemic training failure on mental health and career satisfaction of UK trainees: Lessons from an online attitudes survey. *International Journal of Social Psychiatry,* **55**, 180–190.

Lydall, G. J., & Bourke, J. H. (2009). Rationalising medical careers. *Psychiatric Bulletin,* **33**, 309–312.

Maidment, R., Livingston, G., Katona, C., McParland, M., & Noble, L. (2004). Change in attitudes to psychiatry and intention to pursue psychiatry as a career in newly qualified doctors: a follow-up of two cohorts of medical students. *Medical Teacher,* **26**, 565–569.

Manassis, K., Katz, M., Lofchy, J., & Wiesenthal, S. (2006). Choosing a career in psychiatry: influential factors within a medical school program. *Academic Psychiatry,* **30**, 325–329.

Marshall, M., & Lockwood, A. (1998). Assertive community treatment for people with severe mental disorders. *Cochrane Database of Systematic Reviews,* **2**, CD001089.

McParland, M., Noble, L. M., Livingston, G., McManus, C. (2003). The effect of a psychiatric attachment on students attitudes to and intention to pursue psychiatry as a career. *Medical Education,* **37**, 447–454.

Mickelson, J. J., & MacNeily, A. E. (2008). Translational education: tools for implementing the CanMEDS competencies in Canadian urology residency training. *Canadian Urological Association Journal,* **2**, 395–404.

Mihalynuk, T., Leung, G., Fraser, J., Bates, J., & Snadden, D. (2006). Free choice and career choice: Clerkship electives in medical education. *Medical Education,* **40**, 1065–1071.

National Institute for Innovation and Improvement and Academy of Medical Royal Colleges (2009). Medical Leadership Competency Framework. Health.

Newshound. (2009). Consultant led service not feasible.

NHS Employers. (2008). Medical training and careers – the employers vision. Health.

Rothman, D. J., McDonald, W. J., Berkowitz, C. D., et al. (2009). Professional medical associations and their relationships with industry: A proposal for controlling conflict of interest. *JAMA,* **301**, 1367–1372.

Royal College of Psychiatrists,. (2007). *Fair Deal*. London.

Royal College of Psychiatrists. (2008). *Finding the balance: The psychiatric training value of Out of Hours Working*. London. http://www.rcpsych.ac.uk/pdf/PTC%20The%20training%20value%20of%20OOH.pdf.

Seed, K., Lydall, G. J., Malik, A., Howard, R., Bhugra, D. (2010). *Improving Recruitment to Psychiatry: A Review*. In press.

Shelley, R. K., & Webb, M. G. (1986). Does clinical clerkship alter students' attitudes to a career choice of psychiatry? *Medical Education,* **20**, 330–334.

Starr, P. (1982). *The Social Transformation of American Medicine*. Basic Books.

Thomas, T., & Thomas, T. (2008). Factors affecting career choice in psychiatry: a survey of RANZCP trainees. *Australasian Psychiatry,* **16**, 179–182.

Tooke, J. (2007) *Aspiring to Excellence. Findings and Recommendations of the Independent Inquiry into Modernising Medical Careers.* London: Aldridge Press.

Wallace, E. & Tisdall, G. (1991). Long-term psychotherapy training in residency: Influences on therapy and training. *Canadian Journal of Psychiatry,* **36**, 512–516.

WHO. (2008). mhGAP: Mental Health Gap Action Programme: Scaling Up Care for Mental, Neurological and Substance Use Disorders. Retrieved 6 June 2009 from http://www.who.int/mental_health/mhgap_final_english.pdf.

Wigney, T., Parker, G. et al. (2007). Medical student observations on a career in psychiatry. *Australian & New Zealand Journal of Psychiatry,* **41**, 726–731.

Wright, C., Catty, J., Watt, H., & Burns, T. (2004). A systematic review of home treatment services: classification and sustainability. *Social psychiatry and psychiatric epidemiology,* **39**, 89–96.

Chapter 8

Psychiatry's contract with society: what do clinical psychiatrists expect?

Daniel McQueen, George Ikkos,
Paul St John-Smith, Philip Kemp,
Povl Munk-Jørgensen, and Albert Michael

Introduction

Psychiatry is a complex medical specialty, not uncommonly oversimplified. The importance of families and carers adds a layer of complexity. Different stakeholders bring different expectations. Important stakeholders in third party, state-funded and state-provided mental health services include service managers, service purchasers, politicians, and the general public.

Compulsory treatment is sometimes needed but at the core of psychiatry is the importance of patient choice and recovery and the patient–doctor relationship (Sugarman, Ikkos, & Bailey, 2009). Recently we (McQueen et al., 2009) set out our views about the 7 Es of professionalism (see Table 8.1) and multidisciplinary work in clinical psychiatry. Here we summarize some of the difficulties that need to be understood by stakeholders for clinical practice to be effective. We set out what clinical psychiatry is, including the importance of the patient–doctor relationship, patient choice, and empowerment and multi-disciplinary work. From a position of commitment to this view we identify some other partial conceptions of the specialty which, if applied uncritically, have risks for patients. Clinical psychiatrists expect that all stakeholders in mental health understand the complexity of the specialty and support constructively but not necessarily uncritically, the development and practice of the profession along the lines set out here.

The nature of clinical psychiatry

Medicine and psychiatry developed from concepts of healing and spirituality, which remain at the core of modern professionalism. The practice of medicine

Table 8.1 7 Es of psychiatric professionalism

---
1. *Evidence*: Staying abreast of, and critically appraising scientific developments underpinning psychiatric practice
2. *Ethics*: Applying ethical principles to daily practice: respect for autonomy, beneficence, non-maleficence, and justice; plus concern for their scope of application
3. *Emotion*: Being alert to how emotions of patients and staff interact, including group dynamics
4. *Expertise*: The synthesis of clinical information and scientific knowledge in reflective practice
5. *Engagement*: With service development and leadership
6. *Education and research*: Generating new knowledge and facilitating the acquisition of skills and knowledge among colleagues and the next generation of mental health care workers
7. *Empowerment*: Of patients to maximize their autonomy and achieve recovery
---

and psychiatry requires sensitivity to changing cultures and social expectations. Furthermore, psychiatry is a clinical discipline that relies on scientific evidence.

Psychiatric morbidity in the United Kingdom is approximately 250/1000 population. Mental disorder is especially prevalent in general hospital inpatient and outpatient populations where it is often unrecognized and undertreated (Royal College of Psychiatrists, 2003; Sheehan, Karim, & Burns, 2009). Of the 250/1000 prevalent cases in the general population 230 will consult their general medical practitioner (GP), who will recognize 140 as having a psychiatric condition and refer 17 to psychiatric services, of whom 6 will become inpatients. Thus most of the service needs are in primary care and a small proportion of patients reach secondary care (Goldberg, 1995). Consequently primary, secondary, and tertiary services deal with different psychiatric problems.

Affect, conceived as feelings, emotions, and agitations and manifested in consciousness, behaviour, and relationships in family and society is at the core of psychiatry (Ikkos, Bouras, McQueen, & St Smith, 2010). Affective neuroscience, ethology, and attachment theory show how emotions are the glue of social interactions; from the moment of birth we are instinctually driven to engage with others: The representation of mental states in self and others (mentalization) is vital to affect regulation and effective social adaptation; affect regulation and mentalization are acquired through attachment relationships and contribute significantly to emotional resilience, which helps us weather the challenges that life presents and reduces the risk of psychiatric illness (Fonagy, Gergely, Jurist, & Target, 2004; Sroufe, Egeland, Carlson, & Collins, 2005). Humans are evolved biological organisms; therefore scientific understanding of psychiatric disorders should be rooted in (but not restricted to) the biological sciences (Abed, 2000).

Proximate mechanisms (neurochemicals, hormones, synaptic transmission, etc) are only one aspect of the causation of illness and behaviour. Other individual factors explaining the idiosyncratic expression of both genes and behaviour come from a person's developmental environment, and ultimately the ancestral environment of the species. In humans, environment and personal meaning play central roles. Evolution provides an overarching theoretical framework that permits the integration of these different levels of explanation; nothing in biology makes sense except in the light of evolution (Dobzhansky, 1973).

Diagnosis is essential for communication between clinicians. However, it is only one part of optimal decision-making in treatment or prognosis. Experienced clinicians are aware that diagnosis may stigmatize or have other adverse social and psychological consequences. They rely on a wide array of patient preferences, characteristics, and values in deciding management (Higgins & Tully, 2005). In mental ill health, the clinical picture is usually profoundly shaped by factors specific to the individual and his or her environment. Judgement is required to distinguish abnormal from normal. Individuals vary in where they draw these lines. Social class, education, culture, and beliefs may influence these judgements. The clinical understanding of patients therefore must also be informed by the social and psychological sciences, literature, and the arts and spirituality (Cook, Powell, & Sims, 2009; Oyebode, 2009).

The biopsychosocial model uses detailed empirical understanding of the person's biological endowment, mind, social environment, and their reciprocal interactions to understand mental ill health (Engel, 1977). Psychiatric formulation is more sophisticated than diagnosis. It is a statement of the patient's problem that covers, the predisposing, precipitating, perpetuating, and protective factors in the patient's past and present from biological, psychological, and social perspectives. It may include, where relevant, genetics, life history from conception to the present, insults to the brain and mind, physical and emotional trauma, and psychosocial development including early relationships, current family, work, and social networks.

Producing an effective and efficient treatment plan requires a global understanding of how different factors in patients' lives interact, establishing likely causal relationships between problems, and how health service resources can be deployed most effectively and efficiently. Psychiatrists uniquely are trained to make diagnoses, comprehensive formulations, and strategic treatment plans, focussing on physical, psychological, or social factors, where relevant. Patient values and empowerment are increasingly important.

The importance of patient choice and patient–doctor relationship

At the core of medical activity is the patient–doctor relationship. Patients form attachments to their professional carers, which influence engagement in therapy and outcome. In the treatment of depression the quality of the relationship between patient and clinician has a bigger effect size than the treatment itself, whether medication, interpersonal psychotherapy (IPT), Cognitive Behaviour Therapy (CBT), or even placebo (Krupnick et al., 1996). The strength of patient preference significantly influences whether patients take up treatment and complete it. Research on depressed patients in primary care offered medication or psychotherapy showed that preference in itself influenced whether patients initiated the treatment they were assigned to, whereas strength of preference had a greater effect on both initiation and adherence to pharmacotherapy and psychotherapy (Raue, Schulberg, Heo, Klimstra, & Brice, 2009).

There is a lack of similar research in schizophrenia and other mental disorders. The importance of choice and strength of preference in other disorders may be different. The popularity of the choice agenda and the recovery model among mental health services users and their organizations suggests that preference is of great importance generally. Evidence-based guidelines that ignore the importance of patient preferences may inappropriately restrict patient choice. Even when offered the same treatment the patient may respond differently to different clinicians. One may have the correct model or treatment but the wrong people applying it.

Psychiatrists do not have a monopoly of expertise. Besides fellow professionals' expertise, patients' 'expertise' should be integrated into the process of reaching 'practice/clinical decisions'. Psychiatry requires that the patient–doctor relationship be based on dialogue. Within the context of such a dialogue not only the patient's but also the psychiatrist's (and other professionals') expertise must be recognized and valued. At times of mental incapacity owing to illness, or at times of onset (or possible onset) of new mental ill health, professional expertise, including diagnostic expertise, is particularly important.

Systemic and multidisciplinary issues in psychiatry

The importance of families and carers is difficult to overstate. They provide most of the care and much of the social support that patients receive. They are emotionally involved in ways that are usually helpful and less commonly unhelpful. Their views and wishes may support or undermine patients' wishes or the views of professionals and this can give rise to cooperation or creative tension or harmful conflict. Conflict may be open and acknowledged, covert, or unconscious.

One of the defining characteristics of mental health services is the range of disciplines that frequently need to be involved in the care of a single individual (nursing, social work, occupational therapy, etc). In the United Kingdom, a review of the skills, knowledge, and attitudes required in common by the key professional disciplines in mental health services lead to the framework of capabilities (Table 8.2).

A strength and difficulty for multidisciplinary teams (MDTs) is that the different members vary in their training, professional status, legal authority, remuneration, institutional position and, at an individual level, experience, talent, capacity, and skill. Undoubtedly patients benefit from access to different individuals and the range of knowledge and expertise of the different professions in MDTs. These differences can give rise to cooperation, creative rivalry, or destructive rivalry at the expense of the task of treating patients. On the contrary, the fear of being envied can lead talented individuals to hide their worth and play down their skill, thus depriving the group of their talent (Main, 1975). For barriers to effective team working, see Table 8.3 (McQueen et al., 2009).

The plurality of philosophies of the different professions can support a range of treatments and approaches that enhance clinical effectiveness, efficiency, and patient choice. Equally, different philosophies of care can exacerbate team

Table 8.2 Framework of capabilities

Ethical Practice
The values and attitudes necessary for modern mental health practice
Knowledge
Of policy, legislation, mental health, and mental health services
The Process of Care
Effective communication
Effective partnership with users and carers
Effective partnership in teams and with other agencies
Comprehensive assessment
Care planning, coordination and review
Supervision
Professional development and lifelong learning
Clinical and practice leadership
Interventions
Medical and physical care
Psychological, social, and practical
Mental health promotion
Applications to specific service settings

Table 8.3 Barriers to effective team working

Lack or respect for the team as a group
Lack of investment of team with authority
Lack of clear leadership
Non-recognition of professional values by outsiders
Lack of clarity about objectives
Lack of active participation or focus on team processes (Subgroup rivalry)
Uniprofessional esprit de corps
Interprofessional corridor conflicts
Interdisciplinary suspicion
Lower levels of participation
Working alone or in 'pseudo-teams'
Diverse objectives
Different philosophies of care
Different perspectives on what is judged quality of care
Less stable relationships
High staff turnover
Not valuing the task and quality care
Lower commitment to quality
Lower support for innovation
Individual factors
Poorer mental health in staff
High staff burnout

dysfunction, particularly if individuals or professions adhere rigidly or dogmatically to single perspectives (McQueen et al., 2009).

Rivalry and splitting in teams can also reflect splits in the patient's inner world. The inevitable fact of splitting requires skilful handling to minimize ruptures in treatment and can be turned to therapeutic advantage if the staff team has the capacity and opportunity to reflect regularly on the splits among staff as they occur (Main, 1946). Reflective practice may enhance the functioning of MDTs (Schön, 1983). A unique feature of psychiatry is the influence of our own personal characteristics on diagnosis and treatment (Gabbard, 1999). After evaluation and treatment skills the second most highly regarded skill in psychiatry is the ability to recognize and deal with counter-transference and its influence on interactions with patients (Langsley & Yager, 1988). Failure to do so can have dire consequences (Watts & Morgan, 1994). Open systems theory and psychodynamic models may help understand how conscious and unconscious tensions between groups within organizations can undermine performance of the primary task (Roberts, 1994). The effective support of management in protecting the permeable boundary between the team and the outside world, and ensuring team stability, are essential for reflective practice to occur. Conversely management cultures that tend to favour constant change and/or 'quick fixes' may impede such practice.

Some other perspectives on psychiatry

Psychiatric practice and its priorities may be conceptualized in different ways. We have somewhat arbitrarily grouped some of these into ideological, clinical, and managerial models, which overlap. Here *ideological* does not mean a lack of factual basis rather that some facts have been over-emphasized and others de-emphasized to support a particular viewpoint.

Ideological models that prioritize the wishes of patients include consumer models. These regard patients as rational consumers and the best judges of good care, and consumer choice as promoting quality (Department of Health, 2006; McIntosh, 2009). Some forms of the recovery movement or empowerment model see psychiatrists' function as empowering the 'service user' or 'survivor' to achieve fulfilment in their own terms and freedom from oppression and stigma (Mountain & Shah, 2008). Other ideological models see psychiatrists as agents of political oppression, repressing discontent and other thoughts, emotions, and actions by medicalizing them (Sullum, 2008; White, 2002); or that psychiatrists use drugs to medicate people into passivity and rob them of their individuality, specifically groups defined by gender, ethnicity, or religion. Yet other models see psychiatrists as a self-serving group colluding with the pharmaceutical industry to profiteer at patients' expense (Healy, 2006).

The *medication model* views mental ill health as a biological problem, to be corrected with medication, where the psychiatrist is disengaged from the patient as a person (Bullmore, Fletcher, & Jones, 2009). This is a narrow biomedical model of psychiatry, which some mistake as the dominant model of the specialty. Biological reductionism, the pharmaceutical industry, or economic pressures may drive this model of care (Kontos, Querques, & Freudenreich, 2006). At the extreme medication may be seen as invariably ineffective and harmful.

Economic considerations do not invariably lead to a medication model. Economic arguments have led to spending vast sums of money on short courses of CBT for people with depression and anxiety (which have high rates of spontaneous remission) to return them to productive employment with anticipated net savings to the exchequer (London School of Economics Centre for

Economic Performance Mental Health Policy Group, 2006). Public health physicians, health economists, and the utilitarian approach argue that money is most effectively spent in treating the largest number of people or in preventative measures. Governments in most countries have a determining role in resource allocation. Groups that lobby effectively may gain more resources. Such priorities may differ from those of psychiatrists who may prioritize the treatment of the most acutely or severely ill and disabled.

Managed mental health services have arisen in large part, but not exclusively, out of a need to meet requirements of justice, that is, provide fair access to treatment for all and ensure standards of care for the most vulnerable. This objective is ideal and participation and leadership by psychiatrists in such processes is essential. However, the simplistic pursuit by management of efficiency in such services risks turning patients into objects on a production line where the cheapest labour appears to be most cost-effective, and well-trained highly experienced professionals are inappropriately seen as too expensive. Underlying this is an assumption that patients, with all of their individual and situational differences, can be reliably described by numerical scores for diagnosis, need, risk, complexity, and so on, that can be added together, manipulated statistically, and audited to generate meaningful global figures (Power, 1997).

Recent years have seen a large expansion of managerial staff in UK NHS mental health services. The 'manager/administrator:clinical-staff' ratio increased from 1:15.7 in 2000 to 1:9.7 in 2007 (Goldberg, 2008). The NHS Institute for Innovation and Improvement has been promoting management models that attempt to reduce short-term costs by breaking down psychiatric care into components and devolving them to different teams and team members. However, patients value continuity of care, and it may not be cost effective, clinically effective or acceptable to patients to receive their care from many different clinicians (Dewan, 1999; Goldman et al., 1998).

Increasingly there is a drive to transfer skills to, on the face of it, less expensive staff. This makes intuitive sense, and psychiatrists must engage actively when this is appropriate. However, this may not always be clinically or economically effective. This caution is not unique to psychiatry. For example, a large study showed slightly better outcomes for doctor compared to nurse endoscopies (Williams, Russel et al., 2009). Doctors were more cost-effective because of better outcomes, even though they cost slightly more than nurses (Richardson et al., 2009; Williams, Richardson, & Bloor, 2009). This study shows that even small differences in detection rates can lead to significant differences in outcome and longer-term cost.

Similar comparative research into the assessment of deliberate self-harm (DSH) has shown conflicting findings. One study compared DSH assessment by doctors and nurses using proforma and reported no major differences (Catalan et al., 1980). Another study comparing assessments using proforma by one liaison psychiatric nurse and rotating duty psychiatrists found that the nurse detected more alcohol use. This could result from differences in individual sensitivity, chance, or working hours (Griffin & Bisson, 2001). One study found that social workers were more cautious and more likely to consider that patients had abnormal personalities and physical illnesses, and needed a psychiatrist's involvement or hospitalization. Psychiatrists were more likely to think that patients required help from the local authority (psychiatrists 42%, social workers 7%) and social workers believed that the patient required hospital-based help (psychiatrists 28%, social workers 65%) (Newson-Smith & Hirsch, 1979). Another study compared trainee psychiatrists and psychiatric nurses; doctors were significantly more likely to refer individuals for psychiatric follow-up that involved direct contact with other doctors (psychiatrists 71%, psychiatric nurses 34%). Doctors were also significantly more likely than nurses to perceive individuals as having a mental illness (79% vs. 49%) (Weston, 2003). These differences may have major implications as patients who discharge themselves from hospital after DSH and before completing initial management have a considerably increased rate of repetition (Crawford & Wessely, 1998).

Research comparing professions' ability to recognize psychosis and impaired reality testing found that psychiatrists were more accurate than nurses who were more accurate than psychologists (Nielsen et al., 2008). Professional assumptions and training may empower some and impede others in this area. Further work is required to explore these differences and to obtain accurate role ascriptions.

Conclusion

Psychiatry is devoted to the assessment, diagnosis, treatment, prevention, and study of mental ill health (Marneros, 2008). The complexity in presentation, aetiology, and management of mental disorder is such that no single model can provide sufficient explanation in all cases. Diverse perspectives can enable the clinician to develop a thorough understanding of patients and provide new avenues for research. The complexity of psychiatry is compounded by ambiguity, and psychiatrists have to learn to tolerate this. Eclecticism is a strength and not weakness of the specialty. Multiple viewpoints from different professions can complement each other, lead to creative cooperation, enhance choice, and benefit patients and their carers. On the contrary, adherence to simplistic models and rhetoric can lead to destructive rivalry. Service purchasers and service managers have a crucial role in determining whether teams work creatively to reflect the diversity of the specialty and the needs of patients or get mired in rivalry and dogmatism.

Psychiatrists expect to be held accountable against the complex understanding of the specialty as set out here. Although some members of the profession may fall below the standards implicit in our formulation, the profession as a whole should not be unfairly stigmatized by oversimplistic criticism. Criticism of course is important and critical friends are particularly welcome, but the considerable skills and potential role of the psychiatrist in contemporary mental health services (Bhugra, 2010) should also be welcome and appropriately acknowledged by all stakeholders.

The roots of psychiatry in healing and spirituality and the importance of the patient–doctor relationship must be acknowledged, supported, and developed further through the design of services and the creation of working conditions for psychiatrists that give opportunities for such factors to play an active and beneficent part in treatment and recovery processes. Patients must have opportunities to exercise choice, including the choice to see a psychiatrist and to form a meaningful clinical relationship with her/him. The training of psychiatrists must be effectively supported by curricula, training processes, career structures, and service design and delivery that give real and consistent opportunities for the development and retention of necessary skills and people for the practice of this complex and evolving medical specialty.

Psychiatrists are necessary to provide leadership, synthesize information, and enable teams to work effectively, but leadership is not an exclusive prerogative of psychiatrists. They should actively seek to complement and enrich clinical experience and wisdom with the development and application of robustly evaluated and validated leadership and management skills and activities, and be actively encouraged and supported to contribute to service purchasing and management. They should engage in such positions in a way that appropriately allows the utilization of clinical wisdom and not simply as 'businessmen' or 'managers' manqué.

Acknowledgement

We wish to thank Professors Mario Maj, Professor of Psychiatry, University of Naples and President, World Psychiatric Association and Nick Bouras, Professor Emeritus of Psychiatry, Department of Health Service and Population Research and Director, Maudsley International Partnership Board, Institute of Psychiatry, King's College, London and Drs Lindsey Edwards, Rachael Lippett and Esther Serrano-Ikkos, Consultant Clinical Psychologists, National Health Service, England for helpful comments on earlier drafts of this chapter.

References

Abed, R. T. (2000). Editorial: Psychiatry and Darwinism: Time to reconsider? *British Journal of Psychiatry,* **177**, 1–3.

Bhugra, D.(2010). *Leadership and Excellence in Healthcare: The Role of the Consultant Psychiatrist in Contemporary Mental Health Services.* London: RCPsych Publications (in press).

Bullmore, E., Fletcher, P., & Jones, P. B. (2009). Why psychiatry can't afford to be neurophobic. *British Journal of Psychiatry,* **194**, 293–295.

Catalan, J., Marsack, P. M., Hawton, K., Whitwell, D., Fagg, J., & Bancroft, J. H. (1980). Comparison of doctors and nurses in the assessment of deliberate self-poisoning patients. *Psychological Medicine,* **10**, 483–491.

Cook, C., Powell, A., & Sims, A. (2009). *Spirituality and Psychiatry.* London: RCPsych Publications.

Crawford, M. J., & Wessely, S. (1998). Does initial management affect the rate of repetition of deliberate self harm? Cohort study. *British Medical Journal,* **317**, 985–990.

Department of Health. (2006). *Our Health, Our Care, Our Say: Making It Happen.* London: HMSO. Retrieved 18 June 2009 from http://www.dh.gov.uk/en/Publicationsandstatistics/Publications/PublicationsPolicyAndGuidance/DH_4139925

Dewan, M. (1999). Are psychiatrists cost-effective? An analysis of integrated versus split treatment. *American Journal of Psychiatry,* **156**, 324–326.

Dobzhansky, T. (1973). Nothing in biology makes sense except in the light of evolution. *American Biology Teacher,* **35**, 125–129.

Engel, G. L. (1977). The need for a new medical model: a challenge for biomedicine. *Science,* **196**(4286), 129–136.

Fonagy, P., Gergely, G., Jurist, E., & Target, M. (2004). *Affect Regulation, Mentalisation, and the Development of the Self.* London: Karnac.

Gabbard, G. O. (Ed) (1999). *Countertransference Issues in Psychiatric Treatment.* (Review of Psychiatry Series; J. O. Oldham, & M. B. RIba, series Eds.) Washington, DC: American Psychiatric Press.

Goldberg, D. 1995). Epidemiology of mental disorders in primary care settings. *Epidemiologic Reviews,* **17**, 182–190.

Goldberg, D. (2008). Improved investment in mental health services: value for money? *British Journal of Psychiatry,* **192**, 88–91.

Goldman, W., McCulloch, J., Cuffel, B., Zarin, D. A., Suarez, A., & Burns, B. J. (1998). Outpatient utilization patterns of integrated and split psychotherapy and pharmacotherapy for depression. *Psychiatric Services,* **49**, 477–448.

Griffin, G., & Bisson, J. L. (2001). Introducing a nurse-led deliberate self-harm assessment service. *Psychiatric Bulletin,* **25**, 212–214.

Healy, D. (2006). The latest mania: Selling bipolar disorder. *PLoS Med,* 3, e185. [online]. Retrieved 18 June 2009 from http://www.plosmedicine.org/article/info:doi/10.1371/journal.pmed.0030185.

Higgins, M. P., & Tully, .MP. (2005). Hospital doctors and their schemas about appropriate prescribing. *Medical Education,* **39**, 184–193.

Ikkos, G. (2003). Engaging patients/users as teachers of interview skills to new doctors in psychiatry. *Psychiatric Bulletin,* **27**, 312–315.

Ikkos, G., Bouras, N., McQueen, D., & St Smith, P. (2010). Medicine, affect and mental health services, Commentary on Katschnig, H, are psychiatrists and endangered species? *World Psychiatry*, **9,** 21–28.

Kontos, N., Querques, J., & Freudenreich, O. (2006). The problem of the psychopharmacologist. *Academic Psychiatry*, **30,** 218–226.

Krupnick, J. L., Sotsky, S. M., Simmens, S., et al. (1996). The role of the therapeutic alliance in psychotherapy and pharmacotherapy outcome: Findings in the National Institute of Mental Health Treatment of depression collaborative research program. *Journal of Consulting and Clinical Psychology*, **64,** 532–539.

Langsley, D. G., & Yager, J. (1988). The definition of a psychiatrist: eight years later. *American Journal of Psychiatry*, **145,** 469–475.

London School of Economics Centre for Economic Performance Mental Health Policy Group. (2006). *The Depression Report: A New Deal for Depression and Anxiety Disorders*. London School of Economics, Centre for Economic Performance. Retrieved 20 April 2009 from http:cep.lse.ac.uk/textonly/research/mentalhealth/DEPRESSION_REPORT_LAYARD.pdf.

Main, T. (1946). The Ailment, reprinted in: T, Main 1989. The ailment and other psychoanalytic essays (pp 12-35). London: Free Association Books.

Main, T. (1975). Some psychodynamics of large groups. In L. Kreeger (Ed), *The Large Group* (pp. 57–86). London: Constable.

Marneros, A. (2008). Psychiatry's 200th birthday, *British Journal of Psychiatry*, **193,** 1–3.

McIntosh, K. (2009). Personal health budgets: the patient is always right. *Health Service Journal*, [online] 2 March 2009. Retrieved 18 June 2009 from http://www.hsj.co.uk/personal-health-budgets-the-patient-is-always-right/1988779.article.

McQueen, D., St. John-Smith, P., Ikkos, G., Kemp, M., Munk-Jorgensen, P., & Michael, A. (2009). Psychiatric professionalism, multidisciplinary teams and clinical practice, *European Psychiatric Review*, **2**(2), 50–56.

Mountain, D., & Shah, P. (2008). Recovery and the medical model. *Advances in Psychiatric Treatment*, **14,** 241–244.

Newson-Smith, J. G. B., & Hirsch, S. R. (1979). A comparison of social workers and psychiatrists in evaluating parasuicide. *British Journal of Psychiatry*, **134,** 335–342.

Nielsen, J., Mogensen, B., Martiny, K., et al. (2008). Do we agree about when patients are psychotic? *Acta Psychiatrica Scandinavica*, **118,** 330–333.

Oyebode, F. (2009). *Mindreadings*. London: RCPsych Publications.

Power, M. (1997). *The Audit Society. Rituals of verification*. Oxford & New York: Oxford University Press.

Raue, P. J., Schulberg, H. C., Heo, M. Klimstra, S. & Brice, M. L. (2009). Patients' depression treatment preferences and initiation, adherence, and outcome: A randomized primary care study. *Psychiatric Services*, **60,** 337–343.

Richardson, G., Bloor, K., Williams, J., et al. (2008). Cost effectiveness of nurse delivered endoscopy, findings from randomised multi-institution nurse endoscopy trial (MINuET). *British Medical Journal*, **337,** b270.

Robers, V. Z. (1994). The organization of work, contributions from open systems theory. In A. Obholtzer, & V. Z. Roberts (Eds), 1994. *The Unconscious at Work. Individual and Organizational Stress in the Human Services* (pp. 28–38). London: Routledge.

Royal College of Psychiatrists. (2003). *The Psychological Care of Medical Patients: A Practical Guide, Report of a Joint Working Party of the Royal College of Physicians and the Royal College of Psychiatrists.* College Report 108. London: Royal College of Psychiatrists. Retrieved 18 July 2009 http://www.rcpsych.ac.uk/files/pdfversion/cr108.pdf.

Schön, D. A. (1983) *The Reflective Practitioner. How Professionals Think in Action.* London: Maurice Temple Smith.

Sheehan, B., Karim, S., & Burns, A. (2009). *Old Age Psychiatry, Oxford Specialist Handbooks in Psychiatry.* New York: Oxford University Press.

Sroufe, L. A., Egeland, B., Carlson, E. A., & Collins, W. A. (2005). *The Development of the Person. The Minnesota Study of Risk and Adaptation from Birth to Adulthood.* New York: Guilford Press.

Sugarman, P., Ikkos, G., & Bailey, S. (2010). Choice in mental health, participation and recovery. *The Psychiatrist, 34,* 1–3.

Sullum, J. (July 2000). Curing the Therapeutic State: Thomas Szasz interviewed by Jacob Sullum. *Reason Magazine,* [online] 1. Retrieved 4 June 2009 from http://www.reason.com/news/show/27767.html.

Watts, D., & Morgan, G. (1994). Malignant alienation. Dangers for patients who are hard to like. *British Journal of Psychiatry,* **164,** 11–15.

White, K. (2002). *An Introduction to the Sociology of Health and Illness.* London: Sage Publications.

Weston, S. N. (2003). Comparison of the assessment by doctors and nurses of deliberate self-harm. *Psychiatric Bulletin, 27,* 57–60.

Williams, J., Richardson, G., & Bloor, K. (2009) Study authors respond to editorial. *BMJ,* **338,** b1082.

Williams, J., Russell, I., Durai, D., et al. (2009). Effectiveness of nurse delivered endoscopy: findings from randomised multi-institution nurse endoscopy trial (MINuET). *British Medical Journal,* **338,** b231.

Chapter 9

Teaching professionalism

Richard L. Cruess and Sylvia R. Cruess

Introduction

As physicians recite the Hippocratic Oath or its modern equivalent when they voluntarily join the medical profession, they profess a commitment to a set of ideals and acquire rights and privileges as well as a series of obligations (Kultgen, 1998). These obligations entail both attitudes and behaviours that arise from what it means to be a professional. These obligations must be met if medicine's professional status is to be maintained (Cruess, Cruess, & Steinert, 2008; Irvine, 2003).

Until the latter part of the twentieth century, the attitudes and behaviours necessary to sustain professional status were passed on to physicians by respected role models (Cruess, Cruess & Steinert 2008; Kenny, Mann, & McLeod, 2003; Wright & Carrese, 2001). This system, although imperfect, appeared to work well, but the practice of medicine has changed dramatically by forces arising from within the profession and by changes in society, including health care systems. Teaching professionalism by role modelling depended upon a fairly homogeneous physician population with shared common values. This is no longer the case, and it is reflected in the wonderful diversity found in today's profession and, indeed, in the society that it serves. The increasing complexity and cost of health care, the entry of the state and the corporate sector into the medical marketplace, altered expectations of medicine by a better informed public, and, to a significant degree, the application of 'accounting logic' to the practice of medicine have challenged the medical profession (Freidson, 1970; Moran & Wood, 1993; Starr, 1984). Alterations in health care systems throughout the developed world have placed stress on the professionalism of individual doctors and their organizations (Larson, 1977; McKinley & Arches, 1985; Sullivan, 2005). The nature of the stress has varied depending upon the structure of the health care system and the culture of the country involved (Hafferty & McKinley, 1993; Krause, 1995). These changes occurred against the backdrop of a society that had grown increasingly sceptical of all forms of authority, including those based on the special expertise claimed by the professions (Cruess & Cruess, 1997).

In the 1950s and 60s, social scientists, who have been studying the modern professions for more than 100 years, began to document the many failings of the professions including medicine. Their opinions had a substantial influence on public opinion (Freidson, 1970; Krause, 1995; Larson, 1977; McKinley & Arches, 1985; Sullivan, 2005). The altruism of the profession was questioned, and it was claimed that both individual physicians and their associations had exploited their privileged position in society to further their own ends. The many serious failures in self-regulation were recorded, and it was asserted that the medical profession did not consistently address problems of concern to society. The literature of that time actually questioned the benefits of the profession to society.

As the state and the corporate sector came to have more influence on health care, the values that had been espoused by the profession came into conflict with those of the state and the marketplace. By the end of the twentieth century, social scientists, many of whom previously had been critical of the profession, re-examined their position and came to believe that a system that preserved the professionalism of physicians would benefit society (Freidson, 2001; Stevens, 2001; Sullivan, 2005). This endorsement was qualified by a uniform call for a new commitment to professionalism on the part of the medical profession and indicated that for this to occur, doctors will have to understand professionalism and its relationship to society. It became apparent that relying solely on role modelling to transmit knowledge and pattern the behaviours of the professional to physicians was no longer sufficient. What had previously been implicit should now be made explicit.

During the past two decades this has resulted in a broad-based effort to ensure that professionalism is taught at both the undergraduate and postgraduate levels and that this knowledge is transmitted to practicing physicians. Licensing, certifying, and accrediting bodies have all added requirements that professionalism be addressed explicitly during educational and training programmes and that professionalism be specifically evaluated at all levels (Bataldon et al., 2002; General Medical Council, 2006; Liaison Committee on Medical Education, 2007; Royal College of Physicians and Surgeons of Canada, 2007). Although this is still very much a work in progress, a consensus has emerged on the general principles that should govern the establishment of teaching programmes on professionalism.

Background

There have been two major approaches to the teaching of professionalism documented in the literature. One group believes that professionalism must be taught explicitly, stressing the need to define profession and professionalism and outline the attributes of the good physician (ABIM, 2002; Cruess & Cruess, 1997; Cruess & Cruess, 1997; Swick, 2000). Another group has approached professionalism as a moral endeavour, feeling that experiential learning must be stressed and that role modelling and reflection on real experiences should be the main tools of instruction (Coulehan, 2005; Huddle, 2005). Most educators involved in the teaching of professionalism have come to realize that both approaches are required. If only explicit teaching is used, professionalism will remain a theoretical concept and will not become embedded in practice. On the other hand, for generations professionalism was not addressed directly in the medical curriculum. It was assumed that role modelling would suffice, and that students and physicians in training would both consciously and unconsciously pattern their behaviour on that of those whom they respected. The current dissatisfaction of both the profession and the public indicates that this approach by itself does not work as it is apparent that many physicians do not fully understand their professional obligations. There is now a consensus that those espousing both approaches are correct. Professionalism must be both taught explicitly, exemplary role modelling of professional behaviours be provided, and reflection on personal experiences facilitated (Cohen, 2006; Cruess & Cruess, 2008; Fox, 1989; Ludmerer, 1999b).

An important concept that must be recognized by those designing programmes for teaching professionalism is that the learners are adults (Steinert, 2009). Adult learners are different from younger students, being more independent, usually having their self-defined goals and expectations, often using different learning styles. Generally their motivation to learn comes from within. Most adults prefer to learn by experience in real situations, and what is learned often involves material that is being relearned or reoriented. Learning frequently involves changes in both attitudes and skills. Consequently, active participation is necessary, building on previous experiences in a safe and collaborative environment. There are various theories of learning, but situated learning seems the most applicable to professionalism. Situated learning theory states that learning should be embedded in authentic activities that help to transfer knowledge from the abstract and theoretical to the usable and useful. The behaviours and skills to be learned are often context dependent and real life experience provides the method best suited to adult learning (Brown et al., 1989).

Maudsley and Strivens (2004) have stressed the fact that the educational objective of teaching professionalism is the transformation of students from members of the lay public, or non-experts, into expert members of the medical profession. This relies heavily upon a process termed 'socialization' (Fox, 1989; Hafferty, 2003, 2009) that results in students becoming members of communities or cultures that are joined by 'intricate, socially constructed webs of belief' (Brown et al., 1989, p. 33). Socialization is facilitated by a combination of individual and shared experiences. There must be a balance between explicit teaching of a subject, which clearly must be learned before it is embedded, and activities in which the knowledge learned is used in an authentic context (Brown et al., 1989; Ludmerer, 1999b; Maudsley & Strivens, 2004).

Principles

Teaching the cognitive base of professionalism is not difficult. Establishing an environment where the process of socialization in its most positive sense can take place is much more challenging. The following principles can serve to assist those attempting to ensure that learners understand professionalism and that they are properly indoctrinated into the 'unwritten rules of studenthood and medical practice' (Hafferty, 2006). These principles encompass two large areas of activity. First, faculties of medicine associated teaching institutions, and those responsible for training programs must take a series of decisions that will indicate publicly their support for the teaching of professionalism, provide the resources required by the programme, and create an environment that will allow the programme to flourish. Second, a curriculum must be created that ensures that students and residents can be taught and can learn the essence of professionalism.

The principles outlined below are based upon the literature on teaching professionalism and the authors' experiences. Each institution has its individual culture and what works in one may not be suitable for another. Nevertheless, it is hoped that these general principles may serve as a guide for those designing and implementing similar programmes in their respective institutions.

Institutional support

Developing a major programme for the teaching and learning of professionalism of necessity involves a significant change in any faculty, health care institution, or educational programme (Brater, 2007; Fryer-Edwards et al., 2007; Cruess & Cruess, 2009; Smith et al., 2007; Steinert, Cruess, Cruess, Boudreau, & Fuks, 2007; Wasserstein, Brennan, & Rubenstein, 2007). Because this change must affect both the teaching programme and the culture and environment within which the programme exists, the support of those directing medical schools and teaching hospitals is required (Hafferty, 2003; Inui, 2003). The active participation of deans, department chairs, and programme directors is required to send a message that the subject is important. Their support must be manifested by decisions taken: the allocation of space, teaching time, and financial resources (Hafferty, 1995; Hafferty & Franks, 1994; Inui, 2003). Furthermore, the institution's financial and non-financial reward systems must recognize those who participate in concrete and tangible ways. There also should be consequences for those who fail to do their share in pursuing what has been designated as an important institutional objective.

Leadership and the allocation of responsibility

Closely linked to the issue of institutional support is the need to allocate responsibility for establishing and directing a programme for the teaching and learning of professionalism (Brainerd & Bilsen, 2007; Goldstein et al., 2006; Hafferty, 2006; Kotter, 1996; Steinert et al., 2007). The decision as to who will be responsible is of some importance for symbolic as well as practical administrative reasons. Teaching programmes on professionalism cross departmental and disciplinary lines and should be present throughout the continuum of medical education. An individual and/or a committee should be responsible for guiding the design, implementation, direction, and evaluation of these programmes. This task requires a feeling for the internal dynamics of the faculty, a comprehensive knowledge of professionalism based on contemporary literature as well as tact and diplomacy. The leader/champion should command respect, have easy access to senior administration, be provided with adequate resources, and have the skills and knowledge to both create and administer the programme and serve as its promoter.

In addition to appointing the leader/champion, most faculties choose to establish a committee or working group comprising knowledgeable individuals from the academic units where the majority of the teaching will take place as well as local experts on professionalism and its evaluation (Cruess & Cruess 2006; Smith et al., 2007; Steinert et al., 2007). The committee's function is to advise the responsible individuals, participate in planning, assist in the administration, and provide leadership in the locales were the actual teaching and learning takes place.

The environment

The institutional culture can either support or subvert professional behaviour. Medical education is carried out in an environment that is heavily influenced by two quite different sets of forces, each of which can either support the development and maintenance of professional behaviour in students, trainees, or physicians or actually discourage their emergence. The first, over which educational institutions have only limited control, is the nature of the health care system within which students and their teachers must function. If physicians are forced to see too many patients, if there is too little time for teaching, if physicians must become entrepreneurs in a competitive system, or if students are exposed to persistent inequities in the system, the professionalism of all will be compromised (Ludmerer, 1999a; Relman, 2007; Sullivan, 2005).

However, teaching institutions do have an indigenous environment that they themselves can control. This environment has been analysed in terms of its impact on teaching and learning (Hafferty, 2003; Innui, 2003). There is a 'formal curriculum' outlined in the mission statement of the institution and its course objectives (Hafferty, 1995; Hafferty & Franks, 1994). This states what the faculty believes they are teaching. There is also an extremely powerful 'informal curriculum' consisting of unscripted, unplanned, and highly interpersonal forms of teaching and learning that take place among and between faculty and students. Teachers and role models at several levels, from peers to senior physicians, participate at this level and can have a profound effect for good or ill on the attitudes of students and residents. In addition, there is a set of influences that is largely hidden that function at the level of the organizational structure and culture. The influence of this 'hidden curriculum' on professional values can be positive or very negative. A milieu where poor patient care is accepted or unethical lapses are overlooked as well as decisions that favour research or profit over teaching or ignore patient or community needs sends a message that is difficult to counteract. The informal and hidden curricula are partly responsible for the difference between what students are taught and what they actually learn (Hafferty, 2003). A broadly based faculty development programme can help to change the environment and affect the informal curriculum (Steinert, Cruess, Cruess, & Snell, 2005; Steinert et al., 2007). However, the hidden curriculum also requires attention (Hafferty, 1995; Innui, 2003; Suchman et al. 2004). The incentives and disincentives built into any institutional culture may require changes, along with other factors including economic and structural policies established at the institutional level.

The cognitive base

Students and residents must understand the nature of professionalism, its historical roots and evolution, why the professions are useful to society, the obligations necessary to sustain professional status, and the importance of professionalism to medicine's social contract with society (Cruess & Cruess, 2008; Sullivan, 2005, Wynia, 2008).

The definition and description of professionalism are of paramount importance as they dictate what will be taught, evaluated, and expected of students, trainees, and physicians. Therefore each institution must agree on the substance of the cognitive base, and this should remain consistent throughout the educational process. There is now a rich literature containing acceptable definitions that are available to those designing new programmes (ABIM, 2002; Inui, 2003; Cruess, Johnston, & Cruess 2004; Royal College of Physicians of London, 2005; Swick, 2000). These definitions outline the nature of professionalism and its characteristics. Linking professionalism to the social contract introduces the concept of reciprocity. Individual physicians and the medical profession are granted rights and privileges on the understanding that they will serve society. This 'bargain' (Klein, 1995) outlines the expectations of the medical profession and of society and is therefore the basis of the obligations, 'each to the other' (Cruess & Cruess 2008). If either party fails to meet the legitimate expectations of the other, the social contract will change. Many of the recent changes in the United Kingdom represent a change in the social contract and medicine's professional status. As a result of societal dissatisfaction with the results of medicine's lapses in self-regulation, significant regulatory powers were withdrawn from the profession. This demonstrates a classic cause and effect where the social contract is renegotiated because of the failure of one party to the contract. As professionalism is the basis of this social contract, it also changes when the contract is altered.

There is some evidence that both medicine and society cling to a vision of the professionalism of yesteryear, where physicians were highly trusted practitioners with almost unlimited autonomy. This has been termed 'nostalgic professionalism' (Castellani & Hafferty, 2006). Students, trainees, and practicing physicians must be aware of the evolution of professionalism and of the nature of the 'new professionalism' in which there is increased responsibility to society, more accountability, and more transparency (Irvine 1999, 2007; Royal College of Physicians of London, 2005). This type of social contract better meets contemporary societal expectations.

Professionalism will be taught to individuals with different levels of experience in medicine and in medical schools that use different means of organizing their courses of instruction. The cognitive base of professionalism and its values, attitudes, and behaviours do not change. It is the same for a student, a resident, or a practicing physician and the cognitive base remains constant whether it is taught in a traditional curriculum or in one organized around problem-based learning.

Experiential learning and reflection

Professional identity arises 'from a long term combination of experience and reflection on experience' (Hilton & Slotnick, 2005, p. 63). A major objective of medical education should be to provide stage-appropriate opportunities for gaining experience (Dreyfus & Dreyfus, 1980; Leach, 2002).

Participating in the clinical care of patients has been the most common and the most powerful method of acquiring experiential learning, a situation that has been true throughout the centuries. Exposure to a wide variety of patients and diseases remains the backbone of medical education. However, it will never be possible for a physician in training to see or experience all diseases or the wide variety of ways in which patients present themselves. The use of case vignettes and case presentations, video presentations, and various types of simulations can greatly expand the opportunities for learning at all levels (Steinert, 2009). This is particularly true for the teaching of professionalism as students are unlikely to be exposed to personal experiences involving the many dilemmas faced in practice. Issues involving the role of individual physicians in self-regulation, conflicts between the need for altruism and a healthy lifestyle, the need to fulfil one's fiduciary responsibility to patient's while being conscious of the impact of one's decision on the rest of society can all be faced and discussed in a supportive environment prior to entering practice. For this to occur, those designing and implementing programmes on teaching professionalism must recognize the need and take the opportunity to respond with a formal structured plan to ensure that each student or resident has been exposed to as broad a range of experiences as possible.

A major objective of medical education should not be just to provide stage-appropriate opportunities for gaining experience. It is essential that learners reflect upon these experiences and embed them in their practice (Leach, 2004; Novak, Epstein, & Paulsen 1999). There must be structured opportunities allowing students, residents, and indeed practitioners, to discuss professional issues in a safe environment, personalize them, and hopefully internalize appropriate values and behaviours over the course of education and training (Albanese, 2006; Baerstein & Fryer-Edwards, 2003; Benbasset & Baumal, 2005; Cohen, 2006; Coulehan, Williams, Van McCrary, & Belling, 2003; Cruess & Cruess, 2006; Epstein, 1999; Larkin, 2003; Inui, 2003; Mamede & Schimdt, 2004; Maudsley & Strivens, 2000; Sobral, 2005; Wear & Castellani, 2002). In this way individuals develop their professional identity over time, changing from novices into skilled professionals.

The challenge in designing a programme on teaching professionalism is to ensure that learners at all levels relate their experiences to professionalism and reflect upon these experiences in the context of medical professionalism. The objectives are twofold. The first is for professional behaviour to 'become manifest in lived experiences of physicians' (Coulehan, 2005, p. 893). This is an important part of the process of socialization where the impetus for professional behaviour comes from within the individual (Hafferty, 2003, 2009).The second objective is to have the learners reflect upon the many challenges to their professionalism, which they will face as they function in today's complex health care systems. This should allow them to develop and articulate their own personal attitudes and behaviours in situations involving conflicting values and obligations and to do so in a safe and supportive environment.

There is a large literature on reflection and 'mindfulness' (Baerstein & Fryer-Edwards, 2003; Branch et al., 2001; Coulehan et al., 2003, 2005; Dobie, 2007; Epstein, 1999; Hilton & Slotnik, 2005; Huddle, 2005; Inui, 2003; Larkin, 2003; Novak et al., 1999; Schon, 1987 Suchman et al., 2004; Swick, 2007). Virtually all observers stress the importance of highly personal activities, a safe environment, and interaction between individuals, either on a one-on-one basis or in small groups facilitated by a respected role model. Each faculty or teaching institution must decide the methods that best suit its culture and its resources. The methods available include discussions of meaningful personal experiences in medicine, the use of vignettes, discussion of literature or films, the production and analysis of narratives, organized advisory groups, tutorials, mentors, portfolios in a variety of forms, an analysis of critical incidents, morning report and sign-out rounds, courses in the humanities, events drawn from community service, inter-professional teaching sessions, or any other strategy that can lead a learner to examine his or her responses to dilemmas or difficult situations (Albanese, 2006; Baerstein & Fryer-Edwards, 2003; Branch et al., 2001; Cohen, 2006; Coulehan, 2005; Dobie, 2007; Epstein, 1999; Goldstein et al., 2006; Grant, Kinnersley, Metcalf, Pill, & Houston, 2006; Huddle, 2005; Larkin, 2003; Novak et al., 1999; Suchman et al., 2004).

Structured activities should be planned so that students and residents will, during the course of their reflection, address the major causes of tension that arise at the interface between medicine and society. Thus altruism, lifestyle issues, the role of the individual in self-regulation, conflicts of interest, end-of-life issues, ethical concerns as well as the traditional role of the healer must be included. The importance of medicine as a moral endeavour should be stressed and, although there are clearly situations for which there is no satisfactory answer, issues of right and wrong must be included (Coulehan, 2005; Huddle, 2005).

The capacity for self-reflection of a final year student will be greater than that of one in the first year because of the experiential learning that they have acquired (Hilton & Slotnik, 2005; Inui, 2003; Maudsley & Strivens, 2000). Therefore the activities devoted to self-reflection should be different depending upon the stage of training and should wherever possible be context specific, relating to activities which are taking place at that stage (Ginsberg et al., 2000).

Although all aspects of a programme on teaching professionalism are important, those devoted to providing experiential learning and reflection upon what has been experienced pose the greatest challenge and should be given the highest priority.

Continuity

As increased emphasis has been placed upon the teaching of professionalism, it has become apparent to virtually all observers that professionalism must be taught in an integrated fashion throughout the undergraduate and postgraduate curriculum (Christiansen et al., 2007; Cohen, 2006; Cruess & Cruess, 2003, 2006; Dobie, 2007; Fryer-Edwards et al., 2007; Goldie et al., 2007; Hilton & Slotnik, 2005; Inui, 2003; Kalet et al., 2007; Maudsley & Strivens, 2000; Rudy, Elam, & Griffith, 2001; Suchman et al., 2004; Wasserstein et al., 2007; Wear & Castellani, 2002). The literature is quite consistent, indicating that those faculties of medicine reporting on their experiences have chosen to give a longitudinal course with major components being present during each year of instruction. As the objective is to teach the cognitive base and to internalize the values of the profession, both formal instruction and opportunities for experiential learning and self-reflection appropriate to the stage of training should be provided in all major teaching units. In this way the growth of both explicit and tacit knowledge of professionalism will take place in parallel with growth of knowledge in other areas. Professionalism must be a part of all of medicine and taught in an integrated fashion.

There are two reasons why it is not sufficient to provide opportunities for learning the cognitive base only as an introductory learning experience. First, the professionalism that can be learned by students in the first year is less sophisticated and nuanced than that which can be presented during the final two years when the complexities of the relationships between physicians and patients and between medicine and society are grounded in personal experience. Second, students at all levels should be constantly reminded of the nature of professionalism and of its importance to medicine.

Role modelling

Role modelling remains fundamental to ensuring that the values associated with professionalism will be passed on from generation to generation. Therefore, all teaching programmes devoted to this objective must examine the performance of their faculty members and ensure that they understand contemporary professionalism and model it. Historically, physicians have patterned their activities on those of practitioners whom they respect and trust. Indeed, in times past when most physicians joined the profession by apprenticing to a colleague, role modelling was virtually the only method of acquiring the necessary knowledge and skills (Bonner, 1995; Ludmerer, 1985).

Although this is no longer true, role models remain the most potent means of transmitting those intangibles that have been called the art of medicine (Hafferty, 2003; Huddle, 2005; Kenny et al., 2003; Wright & Carrese, 2001; Wright, Kern, Kolodner, Howard, & Brancati, 1998). They are also important in the development of the sense of collegiality that serves to obtain agreement on the common goals of the profession and encourage compliance with them (Ihara, 1988).

Role models have been defined as 'individuals admired for their ways of being and acting as professionals' (Cote & Leclere, 2000), a definition that stresses their importance to the education of physicians on professionalism. The peer pressure of respected role models remains an enormously powerful tool (Schon, 1987). Conversely, the destructive effects of role models who fail to meet acceptable professional standards can be equally strong (Feudtner, Christakis, & Christakis, 1994).

Unfortunately, there is incontrovertible evidence that the impact of many role models on students is negative. In a widely quoted study, less than half of clinical teachers were identified as positive role models (Wright et al., 1998). In another, half of the clinical clerks and a third of the residents surveyed felt that their teachers were not good role models for doctor–patient relationships (Cote & Leclere, 2000). The impact of poor role models on the informal curriculum is substantial. Students, whose level of cynicism rises near the end of their undergraduate studies (Coulehan & Williams, 2001), invariably report that they are exposed on a regular basis to unprofessional conduct. The usual refrain is that they are asked to 'do what we say, not what we do'(Coulehan, 2005; Inui, 2003).This represents a major obstacle in teaching professionalism, and it must be addressed (Cruess et al., 2008). Role models must be recognized for their contributions, and there must be both financial and non-financial rewards. Furthermore, their performance must be assessed. If found wanting, remediation, must be offered to assist them in improving their performance. If this does not occur, they must be removed from contact with learners. Finally, the institutional barriers to good role modelling should be identified and removed.

No matter what the future of medical education holds, it will remain heavily dependent upon role models for the transmission of knowledge of professionalism and the maintenance of professional values. Thus this aspect of teaching and learning must be addressed.

Faculty development

Faculty development is an essential part of the successful implementation of any new programme on teaching professionalism (Hafferty, 1995;

Steinert et al., 2005). It has been defined as a planned programme designed to prepare faculty and institutions for their roles (Bland, Schmitz, Stritter, Henry, & Aluise, 1990). The impact of faculty development for professionalism can be felt at several levels (Steinert, 2009; Steinert et al., 2005, 2007). First, it encourages the faculty to have a consistent approach to the teaching of professionalism throughout the curriculum, including the undergraduate, postgraduate, and continuing education levels. It gives them an opportunity to agree on and promulgate the same definition, attributes, and behaviours. Second, it can prepare basic science and clinical instructors to both teach the cognitive base and to learn how to provide opportunities for experiential learning and self-reflection in learners. Third, it can help the faculty to become aware of the great importance of their activities as role models. It can assist faculty in overcoming barriers to good role modelling, providing strategies to improve their performance and help them to become more explicit about what they are modelling. Faculty also will become aware of the fact that no one is always an outstanding role model. Recognizing poor performance often can be a learning experience for both the faculty and students (Cruess et al., 2008). Fourth, having a larger cohort of teachers in both the basic and clinical sciences who are aware of and committed to professionalism can actually assist in changing the environment and culture of the faculty and its institutions. Faculty development can thus be effective in addressing the informal curriculum. Fifth, experience has shown that the strategic use of promoting professionalism can actually stimulate changes in the curriculum. Finally, and of great importance, faculty who have participated in development programmes on teaching and/or evaluating professionalism can serve not just as outstanding role models but also as effective small and large group leaders at all levels.

Implementing a comprehensive programme on teaching professionalism is so dependent upon having an informed faculty who are committed to the project that a structured programme of faculty development is a necessity. However, it must be recognized that if this programme is successful, the impact will be felt much more widely. The programme can help to change the hidden curriculum, improving the teaching environment, and assist in implementing change (Steinert et al., 2007).

Evaluation

It is a well-known phenomenon that evaluation drives learning. Thus it is essential that what is taught be evaluated (Stern, 2005). Evaluation can also change behaviour when the behaviours are under scrutiny. Therefore evaluation is a critical part of teaching professionalism. Evaluation must be done at three levels: students and residents, faculty, and the teaching programme itself.

Evaluation of the professionalism of learners at all levels takes two forms. It is essential to test knowledge of the cognitive base (Cohen, 2006; Cruess & Cruess, 2006; Sullivan & Arnold, 2009).This can be done using conventional means such as multiple choice examinations, written essays, short answer questions, OSCEs etc. Knowledge of the cognitive base should be tested in this way because some aspects of professionalism are difficult to evaluate in any other way. As an example, self-regulation, which is such an important obligation, can only rarely be evaluated by observing behaviours.

A more difficult task is the evaluation of values and attitudes that cannot be done directly (Arnold, 2002, 2006; Epstein, 2007; Stern, 2005). However, it can be accomplished by observing the behaviours that reflect these values and attitudes. This must be done not only on students and residents but the professionalism of faculty members must also be examined if a healthy teaching environment is to be maintained. Unfortunately, there are few validated tools to accomplish this task, although some progress is being made in developing them. Global evaluation forms, critical incident reports (Papadakis & Loeser, 2005), the P-MEX (Cruess et al., 2006), peer review (Arnold et al., 2007; Sullivan & Arnold, 2009), 360° evaluations (Arnold & Stern, 2005, Sullivan & Arnold, 2009), and narrative descriptions of behaviours (Coulahan, 2003; Huddle, 2005) are all available. Evaluation of professional behaviours can be formative, with feedback given at regular intervals. This will help those observed to improve their performance. However, to meet medicine's obligations to society, summative evaluations must be done and recorded on students and residents to assure the public of the high standards of those entering practice (Kirk & Blank, 2005; Papadakis et al., 2005).

Summative assessment of faculty can allow role models to improve and will identify poor role models. When unprofessional behaviour has been consistently recorded, remediation should be offered or the faculty member removed from student/residents contact.

Not to be forgotten is the necessity to evaluate the programme for teaching professionalism (Steinert et al., 2007). As establishing such a programme often entails a change in the culture of normally conservative medical schools, the results must be assessed. The methods used can be borrowed from the world of business that has had extensive experience in this area (Kotter, 1996. The assessment of the learners is fundamental to this process, but patient surveys, peer review, and surveys of other members of the health professional team can also be used. The long-term value of the curriculum can be assessed by following the graduates into practice and determining their performance as identified by licensing bodies and professional associations (Kirk & Blank, 2005; Papadakis et al., 2005).

An incremental approach

Designing and implementing a programme whose objective is ensuring that all graduates at either the undergraduate or postgraduate level understand contemporary professionalism and exhibit the behaviours expected of the good physician is a complicated process. As was outlined, the support of the institutional leaders must be obtained, directors named, a definition developed and accepted, faculty trained, buy-in obtained, a formal programme of instruction developed, opportunities for experiential learning and self-reflection developed, and a comprehensive programme of evaluation established. Although it would theoretically be possible to introduce all elements at once, in practical terms, this is not realistic. Therefore, wisdom dictates an incremental approach, where an overall vision is first prepared using broad strokes. Once this has been accomplished, recommendations for concrete changes can be developed and introduced when they are ready. This generally involves the redesign or reorientation of material already being taught as well as the development of new learning experiences. In addition, organizational changes are frequently necessary as the formal, the informal, and the hidden curriculum are assessed and, where necessary, changed.

Summary

As has been pointed out by the Royal College of Physicians of London (2005), 'Medical professionalism lies at the heart of being a good doctor.' Every institution and every individual who is involved in teaching students, residents, or colleagues has a responsibility to ensure that all physicians both understand what it means to be a professional and demonstrate during their day-to-day professional and personal activities that they are professionals. In today's complex world, it can no longer be assumed that the process of socialization, which is experienced by all physicians, will result in a medical profession that consistently meets the high standards expected by the society that we serve. Undergraduate and postgraduate educational programmes as well as programmes of continuing professional development must teach professionalism explicitly and evaluate learners and practitioners at all levels. Only in this way can the profession fulfil its obligations to society under its social contract. As Irvine has stated, 'everyone is entitled to a good doctor' (Irvine, 2007) and it is the responsibility of medical educators to ensure that this occurs.

References

ABIM (American Board of Internal Medicine) Foundation. ACP (American College of Physicians) Foundation. European Federation of Internal Medicine. (2002).

Medical professionalism in the new millennium: a physician charter. *Annals of Internal Medicine,* **136**, 243–246. (Published simultaneously in *Lancet.* **359**, 520–523).

Albanese M. A. (2006). Creating the reflective lifelong learner: why, what, and how. *Medical Education,* **40**, 288–290.

Arnold, L. (2002). Assessing professional behaviors: Yesterday, today, and tomorrow. *Academic Medicine,* **77**, 502–515.

Arnold L. (2006). Responding to the professionalism of learners and faculty in orthopaedic surgery. *Clinical Orthopaedics and Related Research,* **449**, 205–213.

Arnold, L., & Stern, D. T. (2005). Content and context of peer assessment. In D. T. Stern (Ed), *Measuring Medical Professionalism* (pp. 175–194). New York: Oxford University Press.

Arnold, L., Shue, C. K., Kalishman, S., et al. (2007). Can there be a single system for peer assessment of professionalism among medical students? A multi institutional study. *Academic Medicine,* **82**, 578–586.

Baernstein, A. & Fryer-Edwards, K. (2003). Promoting reflection on professionalism: A comparison trial of educational interventions for medical students. *Academic Medicine,* **78**, S742–S747.

Bataldan, P., Leach, D., Swing, S., Dreyfus, H., & Dreyfus, S. (2002). General competencies and accreditation in graduate medical education. *Health Affairs.* **21**, 103–110.

Benbassat, J. & Baumal R. (2005). Enhancing self-awareness in medical students: An overview of teaching approaches. *Academic Medicine,* **80**, 156–161.

Bland, C. J., Schmitz, C. C., Stritter, F. T., Henry, R. C., & Aluise, J. J. (1990). *Successful Faculty in Academic Medicine: Essential Skills and How to Acquire Them.* New York: Springer-Verlag.

Bonner, T. N. (1995). *On Becoming a Physician: Medical Education in Great Britain, France, Germany, and the United States.* New York: Basic Books.

Brainard, A. H. & Bilsen, H. C. (2007). Learning professionalism: A view from the trenches. *Academic Medicine,* **82**, 1010–1014.

Branch, W. T., Kern, D., Haidet, P., et al. (2001). Teaching the human dimensions of care in clinical settings. *JAMA,* **286**, 1067–1074.

Brater, D. C. (2007). Infusing professionalism into a school of medicine: Perspectives from the Dean. *Academic Medicine,* **82**, 1094–1097.

Brown, J. S., Collins, A., & Duguid, P. (1989). Situated cognition and the culture of learning. *Educational Researcher,* **18**, 32–42.

Castellani, B. & Hafferty, F. W. (2006). The complexities of medical professionalism: A preliminary investigation. In D. Wear, & J. M. Aultman (Eds), *Professionalism in Medicine: Critical Perspectives* (pp. 3–25). New York: Springer.

Christianson, C. E., McBride, R. B., Vari, R. C., Olson, L., &Wilson, H. D. (2007). From traditional to patient-centred learning: Curriculum change as an intervention for changing institutional culture and promoting professionalism in undergraduate medical education. *Academic Medicine,* **82**, 1079–1088.

Cohen, J. J. (2006). Professionalism in medical education, an American perspective: From evidence to accountability. *Medical Education,* **40**, 607–617.

Cote, L. & Leclere, H. (2000). How clinical teachers perceive the doctor–patient relationship and themselves as role models. *Academic Medicine,* **75**, 1117–1124.

Coulehan, J. (2005). Today's professionalism: engaging the mind but not the heart. *Academic Medicine,* **80**, 890–898.

Coulehan, J., & Williams, P.C. (2001). Vanquishing virtue: The impact of medical education. *Academic Medicine,* **76**, 598–605.

Coulehan, J., Williams, P., Van McCrary, S., & Belling, C. (2003). The best lack all conviction: Biomedical ethics, professionalism, and social responsibility. *Cambridge Quarterly. Health Care Ethics,* **12**, 21–38.

Cruess, R. L., & Cruess, S. R. (1997). Teaching professionalism in the service of healing. *Academic Medicine,* **72**, 941–952.

Cruess, S. R. & Cruess, R. L. (1997). Professionalism must be taught. *BMJ,* **7123**, 1674–1677.

Cruess, S. R., Johnston, S., & Cruess, R. L. (2004). Profession, a working definition for medical educators. *Teaching and Learning in Medicine,* **16**, 74–76.

Cruess, R. L., Herold-McIlroy, J., Cruess, S. R., Ginsberg, S., & Steinert, Y. (2006). The P-MEX (Professionalism Mini Evaluation Exercise): A preliminary investigation. *Academic Medicine (RIME Supplement),* **81**, S74–S79.

Cruess, R., & Cruess, S. (2006). Teaching Professionalism: General principles. *Medical Teacher,* **28**, 205–208.

Cruess, R. L. & Cruess, S. R. (2008). Expectations and obligations: professionalism and medicine's social contract with society. *Perspectives in Medicine & Biology,* **51**, 579–598.

Cruess, S. R., Cruess, R. L., & Steinert, Y. (2008). Role modeling: making the most of a powerful teaching strategy. *BMJ,* **336**, 718–721.

Cruess, R. L. & Cruess, S. R. (2009). Principles for designing a program for the teaching and learning of professionalism at the undergraduate level. In R. L. Cruess, S. R. Cruess, & Y. Steinert (Eds), *Teaching Medical Professionalism* (pp.73–92).Cambridge University Press.

Cruess S. R. & Cruess R. L. (2009). The cognitive base of professionalism. In R. L. Cruess, S. R. Cruess, & Y. Steinert (Eds), *Teaching Medical Professionalism* (pp. 7–31). Cambridge University Press.

Dobie, S. (2007). Reflections and on a well traveled-path: self-awareness, mindful practice, and relationship- centered care as foundations for medical education. *Academic Medicine,* **82**, 422–427.

Dreyfus, H. L., & Dreyfus, S. E. A five stage model of the mental activities involved in directed skill acquisition. Unpublished manuscript supported by the Air Force Office of Scientific Research under contract F49620-79-C-0063 with the University of California, Berkeley.

Epstein, R. M. (1999). Mindful practice. *JAMA,* **282**, 833–839.

Epstein, R. M. (2007). Assessment in medical education. *NEJM,* **356**, 387–396.

Feudtner, C., Christakis, D. A. & Christakis, N. A. (1994). Do clinical clerks suffer ethical erosion? Student perceptions of their ethical environment and personal development. *Academic Medicine,* **69**, 670–679.

Fox, R. C. (1989). *Sociology of Medicine: A Participant Observer's View.* Englewood Cliffs, NJ: Prentice Hall.

Freidson, E. (1970). *Professional Dominance: The Social Structure of Medical Care.* Chicago: Aldine.

Freidson, E. (2001). *Professionalism: The Third Logic*. Chicago: University of Chicago Press.

Fryer-Edwards, K., Van Eaton, E., Goldstein, E. A., et al. (2007). Overcoming institutional challenges through continuous professional improvement: The University of Washington Experience. *Academic Medicine*, **82**, 1073–1078.

General Medical Council. (2006). *Good Medical Practice*. London: Author.

Ginsburg, S., Regehr, G., Hatala, R., et al. (2000). Context, conflict, and resolutions: A new conceptual framework for evaluating professionalism. *Academic Medicine*, **75**, (10 suppl); 96–511.

Goldie, J. (2008). Integrating professionalism teaching into undergraduate medical teaching in the UK setting. *Medical Teacher*, **30**, 513–527.

Goldstein, E. A., Maestas, R. R., Fryer-Edwards, K., et al. (2006). Professionalism in medical education: an institutional challenge. *Academic Medicine*, **81**, 871–876.

Grant, A., Kinnersley, P., Metcalf, E., Pill, R., & Houston, H. (2006). Students' views of reflective learning techniques: An efficacy study at a UK medical school. *Medical Education*, **40**, 288–290.

Hafferty, F. W. (1998). Beyond curriculum reform: Confronting medicine's hidden curriculum. *Academic Medicine*, **73**, 403–407.

Hafferty, F. W. (2003). Reconfiguring the sociology of medical education: emerging topics and pressing issues. In C. E. Bird, P. Conrad, & A. M. Fremont (Eds), *Handbook of Medical Sociology* (5th ed) (pp. 238–257). Upper Saddle River, NJ: Prentice Hall.

Hafferty, F. W. (2006). Professionalism-the next wave. *NEJM*. **355**, 2151–2152.

Hafferty, F. W. (2009). Professionalism and the socialization of medical students. In R. L. Cruess, S. R. Cruess, & Y. Steinert (Eds), *Teaching Medical Professionalism* (pp. 53–73). New York: Cambridge University Press.

Hafferty, F. W., & Franks, R. (1994). The hidden curriculum, ethics teaching, and the structure of medical education. *Academic Medicine*, **69**, 861–871.

Hafferty, F. W., & McKinley, J. B. (1993). *The Changing Medical Profession: An International Perspective*. Oxford: Oxford University Press.

Hilton, S.R., & Slotnick, H. B. (2005). Proto-professionalism: how professionalization occurs across the continuum of medical education. *Medical Education*, **39**, 58–65.

Huddle, T. S. (2005). Teaching professionalism: is medical morality a competency? *Academic Medicine*, **80**, 885–891.

Ihara, C. K. (1988). Collegiality as a professional virtue. In A. Flores (Ed), *Professional Ideals* (pp. 56–65). Belmont, CA: Wadsworth

Inui, T. S. (2003). *A Flag in the Wind: Educating for Professionalism in Medicine*. Washington DC: Association of American Medical Colleges.

Irvine, D. (1999). The performance of doctors: The new professionalism. *Lancet*, **353**, 1174–1177.

Irvine, D. (2003). *The Doctor's Tale: Professionalism and Public Trust*. Abington, UK: Radcliffe Medical Press.

Irvine, D. (2007). Everyone is entitled to a good doctor. *MJA*, **186**, 256–261.

Kalet, A. L., Sanger, J., Chase, J., et al. (2007). Promoting professionalism through an online professional development portfolio: Successes, joys, and frustrations. *Academic Medicine*, **82**, 1065–1072.

Kenny, N. P., Mann, K. V. & MacLeod, H. M. (2003). Role modeling in physicians' professional formation: reconsidering an essential but untapped educational strategy. *Academic Medicine,* **78**, 1203–1210.

Kirk, L. M. & Blank, L. L. (2005). Professional behavior – a learner's permit for licensure. *NEJM,* **353**, 2709–2711.

Klein, R. (1995). *The New Politics of the National Health Service* (3rd ed). Harlow, UK: Longmans.

Kotter, J. P. (1996). *Leading Change.* Boston, Mass: Harvard Business School Press.

Krause, E. (1996). *Death of the Guilds: Professions, States and the Advance of Capitalism,* (1930) to the Present. New Haven: Yale University Press.

Kultgen, J. H. (1998). *Ethics and Professionalism.* Philadelphia: University of Pennsylvania Press.

Larkin, G. L. (2003). Mapping, modeling, and mentoring: charting a course for professionalism in graduate medical education. *Cambridge Quarterly of Health Care Ethics.* **12**, 167–177.

Larson, M. (1997). *The Rise of Professionalism: A Sociological Analysis.* Berkeley, CA: University of California Press.

Liaison Committee on Medical Education. (2007). *Functions and Structure of a Medical School: Standards for Accreditation of Medical Education Programs Leading to the M.D. Degree.* Washington: Liaison Committee on Medical Education.

Leach, D. C. (2002). Competence is a habit. *JAMA,* **287**, 243–244.

Leach, D. C. (2004). Professionalism: The formation of physicians. *American Journal of Bioethics,* **4**, 11–12.

Ludmerer, K. M. (1999a). *Time to Heal.* Oxford: Oxford University Press.

Ludmerer, K. M. (1999b). Instilling professionalism in medical education. *JAMA,* **282**, 881–882.

Mamede, S. & Schmidt, H. G. (2004). The structure of reflective practice in medicine. *Medical Education,* **38**, 1302–1308.

Maudsley, G. & Strivens, J. (2000). Promoting professional knowledge, experiential learning, and critical thinking for medical students. *Medical Education,* **34**, 535–544.

McKinley, J. B. & Arches, J. (1985). Toward the proletarianization of physicians. *International Journal of Health Services,* **15**, 161–195.

Moran, M., & Wood, B. (1999). *States, Regulation and the Medical Profession.* Buckingham: Open University Press.

Novak, D. H., Epstein, R. M., & Paulsen, R. H. (1999). Toward creating physician-healers: fostering medical students' self-awareness, personal growth, and well-being. *Academic Medicine,* **74**, 516–520.

Papadakis, M., & Loeser, H. (2005). Using critical incident reports and longitudinal observations to assess professionalism. In D. T. Stern (Ed), *Measuring Medical Professionalism* (pp. 159–175). New York: Oxford University Press.

Papadakis, M. A., Arnold, G. K., Blank, L. L., Holmboe E. S., & Lipner R. S. (2008). Performance during internal medicine residency training and subsequent disciplinary action by state licensing boards. *Annals of Internal Medicine,* **148**, 869–876.

Papadakis, M. A., Teharani, A., Banach, M. A., et al. (2005). Disciplinary action by medical boards and prior behavior in medical school. *NEJM,* **353**, 2673–2682.

Relman, A. S. (2007). Medical professionalism in a commercialized health care market. *JAMA*, **298**, 2668–2670.

Royal College of Physicians of London. (2005). *Doctors in Society: Medical Professionalism in a Changing World*. London: Royal College of Physicians of London.

Royal College of Physicians and Surgeons of Canada. (2007). The CanMeds Roles Framework, 2005. Retrieved 5 February 2007 from http://rcpsc.medil.org.canmeds/index.php.

Rudy, D. W., Elam, C. L., & Griffith, C. H. (2001). Developing a stage-appropriate professionalism curriculum. *Academic Medicine*, **76**, 503.

Schon, D. A. (1983). *The Reflective Practitioner: How Professionals Think in Action*. New York: Basic Books.

Schon, D.A. (1987). *Educating the Reflective Practitioner: Toward a New Design for Teaching and Learning in the Professions*. San Francisco: Jossey-Bass.

Smith, K. L., Saavedra, R., Raeke, J. L., & O'Donell, A. A. (2007). The journey to creating a campus-wide culture of professionalism. *Academic Medicine*, **82**, 1015–1021.

Sobral, D. T. (2005). Medical students' mindset for reflective learning: A revalidation study of the reflection-in-learning scale. *Advances in Health Sciences Education*, **10**, 303–314.

Starr, P. (1982). *The Social Transformation of American Medicine*. New York: Basic Books.

Steinert, Y. (2009). Educational theory and strategies for teaching and learning professionalism. In R. L.Cruess, S. R. Cruess, & Y. Steinert (Eds), *Teaching Medical Professionalism*(pp. 31–53). Cambridge University Press.

Steinert, Y., Cruess, S. R., Cruess, R. L., & Snell, L. (2005). Faculty development for teaching and evaluating professionalism: from program design to curricular change. *Medical Education*, **39**, 127–136.

Steinert, Y., Cruess, R. L., Cruess, S. R., Boudreau, J. D., & Fuks, A. (2007). Faculty development as an instrument of change: a case study on teaching professionalism. *Academic Medicine*, **82**, 1065–1067.

Stern, D. T. (Ed). (2005). *Measuring Medical Professionalism*. New York: Oxford University Press.

Stevens, R. (2001). Public roles for the medical profession in the United States: Beyond theories of decline and fall. *Milbank Quarterly*, **79**, 327–353.

Suchman, A. L., Williamson, P. R., Litzelman, D. K., Frankel, R. M., Mossbarger, D. L., Innui T. S. & the Relationship-centered Care Initiative Discovery Team. (2004). Toward an informal curriculum that teaches professionalism. Transforming the social environment of a medical school. *Journal of General Internal Medicine*, **19**, 501–504.

Sullivan C. & Arnold C. (2009). Assessment and remediation in programs of teaching professionalism. In R. L. Cruess, S. R. Cruess, & Y. Steinert (Eds), *Teaching Medical Professionalism* (pp. 124–150). Cambridge University Press.

Sullivan, W. (2005). *Work and Integrity: The Crisis and Promise of Professionalism in North America* (2nd. Ed). San Francisco: Jossey-Bass.

Swick, H. M. (2000). Towards a normative definition of professionalism. *Academic Medicine*, **75**, 612–616.

Swick, H. M. (2007). Professionalism and humanism beyond the academic health center. *Academic Medicine*, **82**, 1022–1028.

Wasserstein, A. G., Brennan, P. J., & Rubenstein, A. H. (2007). Institutional leadership and faculty response: fostering professionalism at the University of Pennsylvania School of Medicine. *Academic Medicine,* **82**, 1049–1056.

Wear, D., & Castellani, B. (2002). The development of professionalism: curriculum matters. *Academic Medicine,* **75**, 602–611.

Wright, S. M., Kern, D. E., Kolodner, K., Howard, D. M., & Brancati, F. L. (1998). Attributes of excellent attending-physician role models. *NEJM,* **339**, 1986–1993.

Wright, S. M. & Carrese, J. A. (2001). What values do attending physicians try to pass on to house officers? *Medical Education.* **35**, 941–945.

Wynia, M. K. (2008). The short and tenuous future of medical professionalism: the erosion of medicine's social contract. *Perspectives in Biology and Medicine,* **51**, 565–578.

Chapter 10

Medicine's social contract with society: its nature, evolution, and present state

Sylvia R. Cruess and Richard L. Cruess

Introduction

The relationship between medicine and society has never been static but for much of its history the medical profession enjoyed periods of relative stability. However, this is no longer true. Many factors including increased effectiveness, cost, and the potential for profit have given medicine a more prominent and important place in society at the same time as society itself was evolving. As a result, the profession's changing relationship to society has come under scrutiny. Indeed, in the United Kingdom this dialogue is quite active and explicit, (Ham & Alberti 2002; LeGrand, 1997, 2003; Salter, 2001, 2003; Smith J, 2004; Rosen & Dewar, 2004; Royal College of Physicians of London, 2005). It has been stimulated by public dissatisfaction with the medical profession following several high-profile failures to self-regulate (Brennan, 2002; Freidson, 2001; Irvine, 2003; Smith J, 2004; Smith R, 1993; Stevens, 2001). In other countries the approach has not been as focused, although debates over the role of the state or the corporate sector in the delivery of health care cannot take place without touching on medicine's relationship with society as a whole (Blumenthal, 1994, 1999; Krause, 1996; Light, 2001; Kirby, 2002; Romonow, 2002; Stevens, 2001).

As long as both society and the medical profession were reasonably satisfied there was little effort to categorize the relationship in a formal way. This has changed and a variety of names have been proposed to describe the relationship. One approach has been to emphasize the moral nature of the practice of medicine, stressing its historical devotion to commitment and service (Coulahan, 2005; Pellegrino, 1990). Those espousing this view have suggested that

---

Note: This chapter is based in part on work previously published in *Perspectives in Medicine and Biology* (2008). **51**, 579–598.

medicine's relationship to patients and society could be called a covenant (May, 1975; Swick et al., 2006), with no emphasis on societal obligations in return. A much larger group of observers believe that the contemporary relationship is more complex and that it entails defined societal responsibilities as well. They have invoked a variety of names including 'bargain' and 'implicit bargain' (Klein, 1983, 1995), 'compact', 'implicit', and 'explicit compact' (Brownlie & Howson, 2006; Ham & Alberti, 2002; Rosen & Dewar, 2004), 'contract' (Starr, 1984), 'moral contract' (Royal College of Physicians, 2005), and 'social contract'(Cruess, 1993; Inui, 1992; Sullivan, 2005; and others). Those suggesting the different descriptors offer some explanation for their choice but have not based their selection on a historical analysis of the organization of society. Because medicine's relationship to society is believed to be based on professionalism (Freidson, 2001; Stevens, 2001; Sullivan, 2005), most observers have linked the two issues.

There has been a surprising degree of agreement on the fundamental nature of the relationship between medicine and society. Even those who do not feel it necessary to formalize the concept with a name believe that medicine has been granted autonomy in practice, a monopoly over the use of its knowledge base, the privilege of self-regulation, and both financial and non-financial rewards. In return physicians are expected to place the patient's interest above their own, assure the competence of practicing physicians through participation in the regulatory process, demonstrate morality and integrity, address issues of societal concern, and be devoted to the public good (Abbott, 1988; Carr-Saunders & Wilson, 1933; Elliot, 1972; Freidson, 1970; Hughes, 1958; Kultgen, 1988; Parsons, 1951; Stevens, 2001). Although there have been disagreements about the motivation of the members of the profession and the state of health of the 'bargain' (Freidson, 2001; Haug, 1973; Johnson, 1972; Larsen, 1977; Light, 2001; Krause, 1996; McKinley & Arches, 1985), its existence seems to have been accepted as has the concept of a mutual state of 'dependency and obligation' between medicine and society (Klein, 1990).

The term chosen is of some importance as it is desirable to have an agreed upon concept to facilitate discussion between medicine and society across both disciplinary and national boundaries. We support the concept of the social contract as the most appropriate and turn to the philosophers for a definition. We propose an outline of the expectations of medicine and society under the current contract and, finally, examine some of the implications of a contractualist approach.

The social contract: origins and evolution

Social contract: A basis for legitimating legal and political power in the idea of a contract. Contracts are things that create obligations, hence if we can view society as organized 'as if' a contract has been formed between the citizen and the sovereign power, this will ground the nature of the obligations, each to the other'(Blackburn, *Oxford Dictionary of Philosophy*, 1996, p. 335).

Starr suggested that the relationship between the medical profession and society is contractual, indicating that the contract was being redrawn in response to the dramatic changes occurring in health care. The last part of his book can be interpreted as documenting the changes in the contract, 'subjecting medical care to the discipline of politics or markets or reorganizing its basic institutional structure' (Starr, 1982, p. 380), a statement which in retrospect appears to have been remarkably prescient. Subsequently many observers including social scientists (Hafferty, 2003; Pescolido, McLeod, & Alegria, 2000; Stevens, 2001; 1999, 2005), lawyers (Rosenblatt, Shaw, & Rosenbaum, 1997), policy analysts (Iglehart, 2005), bioethicists (Bloom, 2002; Kurlander, Morin, & Wynia, 2004; Williams-Jones & Burgess, 2004; World Medical Association, 2005), and physicians(Barondess, 2003; Benson, 2002; Brennan, 2002; Cruess R, 1993; Cruess, Cruess, & Johnston, 1999; Davies & Glasspool, 2003; Gillon et al., 2001; Gruen, Pearson, & Brennan, 2004; Inui, 1992; Ludmerer, 1999; Rettig, 1996; Smith, 2001, 2002, 2004; Wells, 2004) turned to the historical concept of the 'social contract' as being a useful and accurate description of this relationship.

In the United Kingdom of the relationship between the medical profession and society was discussed in depth during the establishment of the National Health Service (NHS). Klein (1983) used the term 'implicit bargain' in his description of this ever-changing relationship. Under the arrangement the government set a global cap on expenditure, whereas physicians exercised considerable autonomy in the use of resources, an arrangement that lasted until health managers wished to exert tighter control. Although some observers in the United Kingdom referred to the presence of a social contract (Davies & Glasspool, 2003; Smith, 2002, 2004), it is probable that Klein's choice of words influenced other commentators in that country who noted, as had Klein (1995), that the 'bargain' had broken down. One new term that was used— 'implicit compact'—was specifically noted to include doctors, patients, and society (Edwards, Kornacki, & Silversin, 2002; Ham & Alberti 2002; Rosen & Dewar, 2004) and presented the relationship between the parties as involving reciprocity; powers are granted to the medical profession on the understanding that the profession will act in a certain way and address certain issues.

The Royal College of Physicians of London (2005) produced a similar proposal but felt that morality was so fundamental to the practice of medicine that the social contract should be renamed a 'moral contract'. They did not elaborate on the difference between the two.

It is of note that the term social contract also has been used to outline many relationships in contemporary society including those that touch medicine directly: between society and its medical schools (Inui, 1992; Ludmerer, 1999; McCurdy et al., 1997; Schroeder, Zones, & Showstack, 1989); between society and science (Gallopin, Funtowicz, O'Connor, & Ravetz, 2001; Gibbons, 1999; Lubchenko, 1998; Slaughter & Rhoades, 2005); and between universities and society(Kennedy, 1997; Kirp, 2003; Lewis, 2006).

The concept of the social contract was developed by seventeenth and eighteenth century philosophers, primarily Hobbes, Locke, and Rousseau, at a time when most countries were ruled by hereditary monarchs (Bertram, 2004; Crocker, 1968; Gough, 1957; Masters & Masters, 1978). It had two purposes: to provide a historical account of the origin of the state and society as citizens united their individual 'wills', and to explain the nature of the relationship between the state and its citizens. It outlined a series of reciprocal rights and duties as being fundamental to this relationship. The concept of the contract continues to have an important place in current philosophic discourse (Bertram, 2004; Daniels, 2008; Rawls, 1999, 2003; Sachs, 2008). Rawls' theory of justice is a contemporary expression of 'contractualist' thinking, stating that 'those who engage in social cooperation choose together, in one joint act, the principles which are to assign basic rights and duties and to determine the division of social benefits' (Rawls, 1999, p. 10). Rawls postulated that the foundation of such a relationship should be justice based on fairness. Although not classifying health as a 'social primary good', he believed it necessary for individuals to be 'normal and fully cooperating members of society over a complete life' (Rawls, 2003, p. 174) and that this constituted an entitlement to health services, a point of view that has been expanded by Daniels (2008). This provides a contemporary Rawlsian contractarian basis for including health and health care in the overall social contract between society and those governing it.

The philosophers endorsing the concept of a social contract were clear that there was no formal legal contract. However, they justified its use as 'the rights and duties of the state and its citizens... are reciprocal and the recognition of this reciprocity constitutes a relationship which by analogy can be called a social contract' (Gough, 1957, p. 245). Contemporary interpretation of contract theory leans heavily on the idea of 'legitimate expectations' as being fundamental to mutual understanding (Bertram, 2004; Rawls, 2003). In addition, a failure of one party to meet the legitimate expectations of the other has consequences in the attitudes and hence the responses of the other.

The social contract can be regarded as a 'macro' contract including all essential services required by a population, but it has also been proposed that there are a series of 'micro' contracts that apply to individual services while conforming to the 'moral boundaries' laid down by a macro contract (Donaldson & Dunfee, 1999a, b, 2001). Health care could be included in the overall relationship as Rawls and others have suggested, or, given its importance to the well-being of both individuals and society, it could be governed by its own micro contract. It appears to us that this latter approach better describes the reality of the relationship. It has the further advantage of allowing health care issues to be addressed in isolation from other issues in society within the context of an overall macro contract.

Finally, although thus far no one has stated so explicitly, it is obvious that the details of the social contract between medicine and society differ substantially between countries, being influenced by cultural, economic, and political factors. Although there are many commonalities that have been documented, there are also significant differences in the funding and organization of health care (Anderson et al., 2005; Ferlie & Shortell, 2001; Schoen et al., 2004), how professionalism is expressed, and in the expectations of the general public (Hafferty & McKinley, 1993; Krause, 1996; Schoen et al., 2004; Tuohy, 1999; Vogel, 1986). What probably does not differ is the role of the healer, which has been present as long as mankind has existed and answers a basic human need in times of illness (Kearney, 2000). Those elements of the social contract that refer to the healer's role will therefore be relatively constant across national and cultural boundaries, whereas those that refer to how the services of the healer are organized, funded, and delivered will vary (Cruess & Cruess, 1997).

In summary, the majority of those analysing the interface between medicine and society appear to believe that it does entail a relationship involving reciprocal rights, privileges, and obligations. The term covenant, no matter how inspiring or uplifting it may be, misses this fundamental part of the contemporary relationship. Of the terms suggested by those who accept the idea of 'reciprocity', only social contract has a historical and philosophic basis, thus increasing its legitimacy. Although originally conceived to protect both individual citizens and the public from the abuses of authoritarian rule, it now emphasizes the mutual rights and obligations of citizens and those governing them. It is now being used to justify a just distribution of necessary services to citizens. Essentially society, acting through its governing structures, cedes authority to the medical community in return for expected benefits to its citizenry (Slaughter & Rhoades, 2005).

The evolution of the relationship

Until recently, most observers have been content to outline medicine's relationship to society, involving mutual rights, privileges, and obligations, in terms best described as bilateral, even though virtually all recognize the presence of multiple stakeholders in the health care field. There seemed to be an assumption that two major players existed: a relatively monolithic medical profession and society, presumably represented by elected officials. Although this may once have been true, the reality is now quite different.

The medical profession of the twenty-first century differs dramatically from that of the nineteenth when the modern profession emerged. At that time, the profession was unified and national medical associations represented and spoke for it (Elliot, 1972; Freidson, 1970; Krause, 1996; Moran & Wood, 1993; Starr, 1982; Stevens, 2001). Formed in the middle of the nineteenth century, professional associations convinced society that allopathic medicine with its scientific base could best assure competence and the quality of care (Freidson, 1970; Krause, 1996; Rayack, 1967; Starr, 1982; Stevens, 1996, 2001; Torrance, 1987; Vaughan, 1975). They set standards, lobbied for improved care, and enjoyed high levels of trust. Most practicing physicians were members. They also engaged in activities designed to protect medicine's monopoly, diminish competition within the profession, and promote the economic interests of physicians. Nonetheless, society felt that the national associations did not abuse their privileged position. Medicine was dominant (Freidson, 1970; Krause, 1996; Light, 2001; Starr, 1982), and it was clear who 'spoke for medicine' as a party to the social contract.

The growth of specialization compromised medicine's unity (Elliot, 1972; Freidson, 1970; Krause 1996; Starr, 1982; Stevens 1996, 2001) as the loyalties of physicians changed. Most felt more comfortable being represented by their specialty associations, thus diminishing the authority of national bodies. This occurred as medicine was challenged by health care environments described as being controlled by a balance of 'countervailing forces' in which the profession, the state, and the corporate sector are the principle actors (Broadbent & Laughlin, 1997; Freidson, 2001; Krause, 1996; Light, 2001; Mechanic, 1991; Moran & Wood, 1993; Starr, 1982; Stevens, 2001). Medicine was dominant in the contract until the mid-twentieth century (Freidson, 1970). It has since lost influence and the state and/or commercial interests are now ascendant (Freidson, 2001; Krause, 1996; Light, 2001; 1991; Starr, 1982) and will remain so in determining the social contract of the future.

In countries with government-based health care systems, ongoing negotiations between the state and the profession became essential (Broadbent & Laughlin, 1997; Klein, 1995; Krause, 1996; Stevens, 2001; Torrance, 1987; Tuohy, 2003; Vogel, 1986), and some organization was required to represent medicine. In the United Kingdom there are several organizations with mandates to do so, the most important being the British Medical Association (BMA), to which 80% of physicians belong (British Medical Association, 2008).

It is recognized as a union whose activities are covered under the labour code (Hafferty & McKinley, 1993; Klein, 1995). It is responsible for negotiating remuneration and working conditions—the most obvious and important elements of the social contract. The Royal Colleges share some responsibility for self-regulation and the General Medical Council (GMC) is mandated to be the primary defender of public safety and plays a greater role in this respect at a national level than does any corresponding body in North America (Irvine, 1999; Stacey, 1992).

In Canada's federal system health care is a provincial responsibility and most negotiations are carried out at that level. All Canadian provinces have transformed their provincial medical associations into legal or quasi-legal unions or have created new bargaining units responsible for negotiating both financial issues and working conditions (Castonguay, 1976; Torrance, 1987). As a consequence, the Canadian Medical Association (CMA), with no direct role in negotiating for incomes, can speak to issues of national concern, including public policy which of course must embody much of the social contract. The CMA is a credible representative of the profession as a comfortable majority of physicians belong to it (Canadian Medical Association, 2005).

In the United States, there has been no stimulus for establishing a formal framework for negotiations (Laugeson & Rice, 2003; Stevens, 2001). Stevens noted the lack of any concentration of responsibility at the national, state, or local levels for health care and no formal delegation of power to medical organizations in relation to organized payment and service systems (Stevens, 2001). The American Medical Association (AMA) that traditionally spoke for medicine has the structure, including representation from the specialty associations to continue this role. However, its low level of membership and the prominence and influence of organizations representing the various specialties has weakened it (Stevens, 2001; Wolinsky & Brune, 1994) with the result that specialty associations often negotiate independently on behalf of their members. In addition, there are legal impediments to the organization of American medicine for collective negotiations (Hellinger & Young 2001; Rosenblatt, Shaw, & Rosenbaum 1997)and many American physicians feel that unionization, which is found in so many developed countries, is incompatible with the professional role (Cohen, 2000; Brewbaker, 2002). This is contrary to the opinion of observers contrasting Britain, Canada, and the United States who have suggested that clinical autonomy and collegiality are better preserved in countries with national health plans and unions (Hafferty & McKinley, 1993; Tuohy, 1999). Furthermore, physicians' unions are the norm in most European countries, and there is no evidence that the core values underlying their social contracts and practices are different

(ABIM Foundation et al., 2002; Hafferty & McKinley, 1993; Krause, 1996; Samanta & Samanta, 2004).

It is thus apparent that for the majority of countries in the developed world, the presence of a national health system has necessitated the identification of the parties to the relationship and clarified who is mandated to speak for medicine. In the United States one of the consequences of the absence of such a scheme has been the lack of a centralized negotiating table and a spokesperson recognized by both society and physicians as representing the profession.

The parties to the contract

Rosen and Dewar (2004) have analysed the relationships between the multiple stakeholders involved in health care and integrated them around the concept of reciprocity. In redefining medical professionalism they proposed a new 'compact' involving three interlocking societal components. The first group consists of patients and patient groups as well as the 'public', the second of health care managers, the state, government departments, and the European Parliament. The final one comprises the medical profession and 'professional bodies'. There is interaction within each group, and each group has reciprocal relationships with the other two. Each relationship is 'mediated' by the media, the legal system, and the regulatory framework. The commercial sector was not included as a major stakeholder or 'mediator'. We are in agreement with their approach but believe that it does not correctly outline the nature of the interrelationships as it treats the two fundamental groupings of society – the general public and government – as independent entities.

A schematic representation of our concept of the contemporary social contract in health care, including its complex interrelationships, is presented in Figure 10.1 (Cruess & Cruess, 2008).

The medical profession: Medicine is not monolithic. It includes individual physicians and those institutions traditionally mandated to carry out medicine's collective responsibilities (licensing and certifying bodies and educational and training institutions) and their national and specialty associations (Parsons, 1951; Starr, 1982; Stevens, 2001, 2002). The interests of primary care physicians do not always coincide with those of specialists (Abbott, 1988; Starr, 1982; Stevens, 2002) and sub-specialization often results in significant differences between specialists(Stevens, 2001, 2002). Professional associations have been described as representing an elite whose priorities may differ from those of practicing physicians (Freidson, 1970; Starr, 1982; Stevens, 2001, 2002). Thus there is a constant interplay between and among individual physicians and medicine's institutions that must take place if the profession is to develop

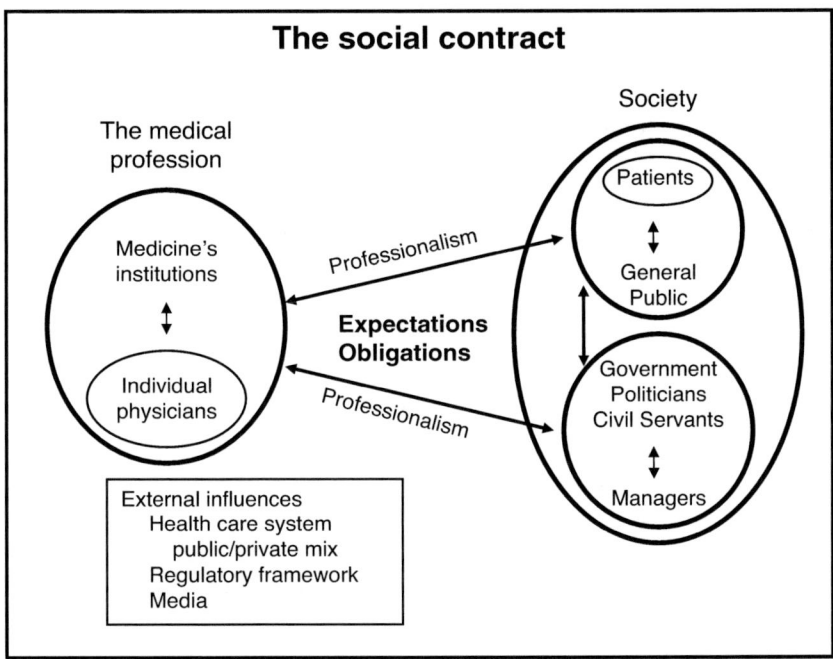

Fig. 10.1 A schematic representation of medicine's social contract with society.

a consensus on the issues pertaining to its social contract with society(Laugeson & Rice 2003; Lewis 2006; Peterson 2003; Salter 2001, 2003).

Society: Society is also complex in a democratic state, consisting of patients etc and the general public on the one hand and government on the other (Krause, 1996; Le Grand, 2003; Richmond & Fein, 2005; Salter, 2001, 2003; Starr, 1982). Physicians and medicine relate to each societal component.

The primary relationship of the individual physician in both moral and fiduciary terms is with the individual patient (May, 1975; Pellegrino, 1990; Rosenbaum, 2003; Rosenblatt, Shaw, & Rosenbaum, 1997). However, this relationship must be seen in the context of medicine's overall relationship with society and cannot be isolated from the system within which it operates, or from the wishes of society as a whole. Other health professionals and their organizations, disease-oriented and consumer groups, industry, individual citizens, and the unorganized general public all are partners to the contract (Blumenthal, 2000; Brown, Zavetoski, McCormick, Morello-Frosch, & Altman, 2004; Callaghan & Wistow, 2006; Ham & Alberti, 2002; Morone & Kilbreth, 2002; Rosen & Dewar, 2004; Salter, 2001, 2003). As is true within the medical profession, there is a dynamic interplay between the various non-governmental stakeholders as they interact with each other, which results in the elaboration of what patients and the public wish from physicians and their organizations (Le Grand, 2003; Morone & Kilbreth, 2002; Salter, 2001, 2003).

In line with contract theory, physicians and those representing them and patients and the general public have expectations, 'each of the other'. A proposed outline of these expectations is given in Table 10.1 (Cruess & Cruess, 2008). Professionalism serves as the basis of this relationship, essentially establishing the rules of the game as outlined in medicine's declaration of applied morality, its code of ethics.

Medicine has an important relationship with the other essential components of society, government also because the profession operates using powers delegated to it by society through government action (Krause 1996; Rosenblatt, Shaw, & Rosenbaum, 1997; Starr, 1982; Sullivan, 2005). Governments are also complex comprising elected politicians, civil servants, and (particularly in publicly funded institutions) managers of the system (Klein, 1990; Morone & Kilbreth, 2002; Rosen & Dewar, 2004; Salter, 2003; Starr, 1982). Again, there is a dynamic interaction between these individuals or groups of individuals that results in public policy. There are also a series of expectations and obligations resulting from the relationship between medicine and government. These are shown in Table 10.2 (Cruess & Cruess, 2008). Because of the current dominance of the state or the commercial sector, to which the state may delegate a major role (Freidson, 2001; Krause, 1996; Light, 2001; McKinley & Marceau, 2002; Starr, 1982; Stevens, 2002), the relationship between medicine and government is now extremely important, as are the expectations and

Table 10.1 The expectations of medicine and patients and the general public of each other

Patients/public expectations of medicine	Medicine's expectations of patients/public
◆ Fulfil the role of the healer	◆ Trust sufficient to meet patient's needs
◆ Assured competence of physicians	◆ Autonomy sufficient to exercise judgement
◆ Timely access to competent care	
◆ Altruistic service	◆ Role in public policy in health
◆ Morality, Integrity, Honesty	◆ Share responsibility for health
◆ Trustworthiness	◆ Balanced lifestyle
◆ Codes of ethics	◆ Rewards – non-financial
◆ Accountability/transparency	respect
◆ Respect for patient autonomy	status
◆ Source of objective advice on health matters	– financial
◆ Promotion of the public good	

Table 10.2 The expectations of medicine and government of each other

Medicine's expectations of government	Government's expectations of medicine
♦ Trust sufficient to meet patient's needs	♦ Assured competence of physicians
♦ Autonomy sufficient to exercise judgment	♦ Morality, integrity, honesty
♦ Self-regulation	♦ Compliance with the health care system – laws and regulations

♦ Health care system
    value-laden
    equitable
    adequately funded and staffed
    reasonable freedom within system
	♦ Accountability
	    performance
	    productivity
	    cost-effectiveness

♦ Role in developing health policy	♦ Transparency in decision making and administration
♦ Monopoly through licensing laws	♦ Participation in team health care

♦ Rewards – non-financial
    respect
    status
    – financial
	♦ Source of objective advice
	♦ Promotion of the public good

obligations of the two parties. Professionalism governs medicine's actions in dealing with governments.

Finally, as society is made up of government and those governed, patients as citizens and the general public enjoy a relationship with government, which is closer to the classical vision of a social contract. Patients, their representatives, stakeholder groups, and the general public must deal with the elected officials, civil servants, and health care managers mandated to ensure that citizens and the public receive the preventive and therapeutic measures in health expected in a modern society (Ham & Alberti, 2002; Krause, 1996; Le Grand, 2003; Rosen & Dewar, 2004; Salter, 2001; Starr, 1982). The expectations and obligations of these parties are illustrated in Table 10.3 (Cruess & Cruess, 2008). Although professionalism does not play a role in this relationship, the nature of the social contract between the public and government is expressed in the structure and funding of the health care system and has a profound effect upon the professionalism of the medicine, either supporting or subverting its healing role and traditional values(Freidson, 2001; Light, 2001; Stevens, 2001; Sullivan, 2005).

The external influences

Three important external influences that have direct and indirect effects on the social contract and on the interactions between the three parties are (1) the

Table 10.3 The expectations of patients and the public and government of each other

The public/patients expectations of government	Government expectations of the public/patients

◆ Quality health care
◆ Health care system
    accessible
    equitable
    value laden
    adequately funded and staffed
    reasonable cost
◆ Transparency in decision making and administration
◆ Accountability
◆ Input into health policy
	◆ Appropriate use of resources
	◆ Reasonable expectations
	◆ Some responsibility for own health
	◆ Support for public policy
	◆ Controlled input into public policy and management

health care system including the role of the private sector, (2) the regulatory framework, and (3) the media.

The health care system and the private sector

The relationship between the commercial sector and both physicians and patients is usually outlined by legal contracts (including insurance policies), not a social contract. However, the role of the market place in health care is clearly part of the overall social contract. Its magnitude is decided by government action (or inaction) and accounts for many of the national differences in the nature of the social contract (Marchildon, 2006; Hafferty & McKinley, 1993; Krause, 1996; Rosenbaum, Frankford, Moore, & Borzi, 1999; Touhy, 1999; Vogel, 1986). Most countries have systems that combine public and private roles, with the decision as to the nature of the mix ultimately determined by legislation. When medicine or the general public wishes to change the system, it must do so through the political process.

The nature of the social contract between medicine and society imposes limits on the legal contracts outlining the obligations of practitioners, the commercial sector, and government. When these limits are exceeded, the public will react. Recent examples include the 'gag laws' in the United States that prohibited physicians from informing patients of therapeutic options not included in their insurance coverage and the attempt to impose a 24-hour limit on hospital stays following obstetrical delivery. The public and the medical profession, supported by the media, objected and, working through the political process, established that some decisions must remain between physicians and their patients (Rosenbaum et al., 1999). There are also limits on the actions of the medical profession. A physicians' strike in Ontario over the right to bill more than the approved fee schedule received no public support. The profession did not gain its objectives and its reputation was severely damaged (Meslin, 1987). These exemplify the often unwritten constraints on all parties to the contract to remain within the moral boundaries perceived to be part of the social contract.

The regulatory framework

The regulatory framework of a country impacts the social contract. Countries such as France, where the government retains the right to regulate, have different contracts from those with systems drawn from the Anglo-Saxon tradition where more emphasis is placed on the independence and autonomy of the profession (Hafferty & McKinley, 1996; Irvine, 2003; Krause, 1996). The recent changes in the governance of the GMC and the allocation of disciplinary power to a new body clearly represent changes in medicines professional status, and in the social contract (Donaldson, 2006; Secretary of State, 2007).

The media

The impact of the media on the social contract can be profound, especially in contemporary society with rapid communication within and between countries. The 'Bristol cases' in the United Kingdom provide a powerful example (Irvine, 2003). Paediatric cardiac surgery was carried out with unacceptably high mortality rates for years. The facts were known to many with administrative responsibility both within and without the institution but it was not until the media revealed them to the general public that action was taken (Irvine, 2003). The result was public indignation and an extensive re-evaluation by government of the concept of self-regulation and recommendations for significant changes in the process including partial withdrawal of the profession's regulatory powers (Salter, 2003; Secretary of State for Health, 2007). The failure of the medical profession to self-regulate constituted a breach of its obligations under the contract and the media was instrumental in highlighting this fact, leading to a change in the contract with an alteration in the expectations of the major parties.

Strains on the contract

For relationships to function properly there must be trust between the parties (Pescolido, McLeod, & Alegria, 2000) and each must not make unreasonable demands on the other (Feldman, Novack, & Graceley, 1998; Freidson, 2001;

Paris & Post, 2000; Salter, 2001). In the health care sector there are many examples where either society or medicine has felt that the other has not met legitimate expectations.

Medicine's failures in self-regulation have been well documented and have led to the belief that the profession is more dedicated to protecting its members than patients (Brennan, 2002; Freidson, 2001; Irvine, 2003; Smith J, 2004; Smith R, 1993; Stevens, 2001). There is also the perception of a decline in altruistic behaviour that has been accentuated by wide public awareness of the presence of serious conflicts of interest (Broadbent & Laughlin, 1997; Freidson, 2001; Jones, 2002; Stevens, 2001). Medicine's associations have come to be regarded as being devoted to the welfare of the profession rather than to the public good (Freidson, 1970; Mechanic, 2004; Stevens, 2001). These issues have led to diminished societal trust, creating tensions on the contract and causing society to modify some of the profession's privileges (Freidson, 1970, 1999; Irvine, 2003; Krause, 1996; Pellegrino & Relman, 1999; Salter, 2001; Starr, 1982; Stevens, 2001; Wolinsky & Brune, 1994).

For their part, physicians feel that those countries using competition for cost control have forced them to become more entrepreneurial and competitive (Krause, 1996; Pham, Devers, May, & Berenson, 2004; Starr, 1982; Stevens, 2001), altering the tradition of collegiality (Ihara, 1988; Parsons, 1939, 1951). Younger physicians feel that the nature of the altruism expected of previous generations places unreasonable demands on their lifestyle (Barondess, 2003; Bickel & Brown, 2005; Blendon et al., 2001; Henningson, 2002; Mechanic, 2003; Smith, 2002). There is evidence that women, who constitute 50% of medical school enrolment, wish modifications to the social contract (Bickel & Brown 2005; Levinson & Lurie, 2004). Many physicians in countries with national health systems such as Canada and the United Kingdom believe that the level of funding of the health care system does not permit them to provide appropriate care for patients (Bloche, 1999; Detsky & Naylor, 2004; Tuohy, 1999; Smith, 2001, 2002). Increasing external regulation and accountability have limited physician autonomy (Blendon et al., 2001; Dunning, 1999; Light, 2000; Morreim, 2002; Smith 2001, 2002; Stevens, 2001; Zuger, 2004) and the growth of medical malpractice claims represents an unwelcome change in the contract (Krause, 1996; Rosenblatt, Shaw, & Rosenbaum, 1997; Starr, 1982; Studdert, Mellow, & Brennan, 2004; Vogel, 1986). The role of the courts in regulating medicine and redefining the legal status of the profession has done much to alter the practice of medicine and the social contract, with the application of anti-trust laws to medicine being a striking example (Krause, 1996; Rosenblatt, Shaw, & Rosenbaum, 1997; Starr, 1982; Vogel, 1986). Finally, physicians recognize that financial constraints, representing contemporary economic reality, often interfere with their fiduciary duty to their patients (Barondess, 2003; Bloche, 1999; Davis & Churchill, 1991; Mechanic & Schlesinger, 1996; Pellegrino, 1990; Stevens, 2001; Tuohy, 2003).

Professional associations, leadership, and negotiations

The profession must assume responsibility for those parts of the contract over which society has granted it authority and over which it can exert control. Assuring competence through open self-regulation is an absolute obligation. Ensuring that the profession understands the necessity for altruistic behaviour and that society believes in its devotion to service is also essential. Those who have approached professionalism as a series of commitments or obligations have urged medicine to meet its obligations and the profession has responded. More rigorous and transparent setting and maintenance of standards and discipline plus enhanced emphasis on educational programmes devoted to professionalism are examples of medicine's response (ABIM Foundation et al., 2002; Accreditation Council for Graduate Medical Education, 2000; Association of American Medical Colleges, 1998; Cruess & Cruess, 1997; General Medical Council, 2006; Irvine, 1999; Royal College of Physicians of London, 2005; Royal College of Physicians and Surgeons of Canada, 2000; Swick, 2000). These efforts, which are of recent origin, must expand and be carried out with rigour.

A different approach must be taken to threats arising outside of the profession over which medicine has no direct control. There is a growing realization that negotiation is an important aspect of contemporary professionalism and that many issues must be addressed in this way (Wynia, Latham, Kao, Berg, & Emanuel, 1999). The social contract, and thus the nature of professional obligations, evolves by negotiations involving all who have a legitimate interest in health care. These take place in a variety of settings and include both financial and non-financial issues. Although some issues are negotiated with commercial organizations, the most important usually involve some level of government.

Rarely has the essential relationship between medicine and society been addressed. A debate did take place in the United Kingdom and Canada preceding the enactment of legislation establishing their national health plans (Coburn, 1993; Klein, 1995; Torrance, 1987). There was discussion in the United States as Medicare and Medicaid were enacted (Freddi & Bjorkman, 1989; Starr, 1982).

Although countries with national health plans are not without problems, a more explicit contract is present, a 'negotiating table' exists, and some organization is mandated to speak for the medical profession. The United States has not developed a forum in which to renegotiate the social contract, and the body with a mandate to negotiate does not enjoy the allegiance of a majority of the profession (McKinley & Marceau, 2002; Wolinski & Brune, 1994). Thus the nature of the social contract in the United States has been shaped by a combination of Medicare and Medicaid regulations and market forces rather than by an integrated series of negotiations.

What is required

If the social contract is to be renegotiated in a comprehensive and coherent fashion, different national strategies are required. Because the profession's status and authority are granted by society, gaining the support of the general public, which at the present time appears to have little input into health policy, is critical (Blumenthal, 2000; Cohen, Cruess, & Davidson, 2007; Davis & Churchill, 1991; Krause, 1996; Mechanic, 2003; Schlesinger, 2002; Stevens, 2001; Sullivan, 1995; Tuohy, 1999). In all countries, issues of importance to both society and physicians must be included, but medicine's emphasis should be on negotiating a health care system, and hence a social contract, that supports, rather than subverts, those aspects of professionalism that are essential for the ethical practice of medicine. This should include the non-financial matters that are of concern to physicians such as patient access and waiting lists, appropriate levels of autonomy, methods of payment that encourage professional behaviour, the proper role of the profession in shaping public policy, malpractice issues, dealing with medical errors, the management of conflicts of interest, the funding of health care, workforce issues, and others.

In countries where mandates and a structure for negotiations are in place, a negotiating strategy should be developed and implemented that attempts to achieve consensus within the profession concerning the nature of the social contract and addresses its elements in a comprehensive fashion during negotiations.

With the current structure of the American health care system, either a reinvigorated AMA or a new body would of necessity be required to negotiate with the federal government over the details of Medicare and Medicaid and with the many players offering health insurance in the market place. At the least, a common set of principles should guide these negotiations, which would include a commitment to structural reform of the health care system. Should some form of universal health insurance result, experience in other countries has shown that this leads to the establishment of either national or regional negotiating tables. These should facilitate the renegotiation of a social contract that supports the role of the healer.

Conclusion

Although society has the right to determine public policy and, once established, medicine must adhere to it, several authors have outlined the advantages to society of negotiating these issues (Benson, 2002; Blumenthal, 1994; Cruess et al., 1999; Freidson, 2001; Hafferty & Light, 1995; Mechanic, 2003; Morreim, 2002; Stevens, 2001; Sullivan, 1995; Tuohy, 2003; Wolf, 1994). As Blumenthal has pointed out (1994, p. 252): 'Health care reform cannot succeed—politically or substantively—unless it preserves and bolsters the professionalism of physicians and other health care providers.' The profession requires the assistance of the political process in maintaining its professionalism (Hall, 2005; Light, 2001).

An essential truth remains: those negotiating on behalf of the medical profession must be seen to place the public interest above their own or it will appear that they are abusing the privileged position granted to professions (Daniels, 1978; Meslin, 1987; Page, 2004). Negotiating responsibly can restore the credibility, legitimacy, and sense of purpose necessary for achieving a social contract that can better serve patients and society while preserving and promoting core professional values.

References

Abbott, A. (1988). *The System of Professions*. Chicago, IL: University of Chicago Press.

ABIM (American Board of Internal Medicine) Foundation. ACP (American College of Physicians) Foundation. European Federation of Internal Medicine. (2002). Medical professionalism in the new millennium: A physician charter. *Annals of Internal Medicine*, **136**, 243–246. (Published simultaneously in *Lancet*, **359**, 520–523).

Accreditation Council for Graduate Medical Education. (ACGME). (2000). *Outcome Project*. ACGME Website. Retrieved 2 July 2010 from http://www.acgme.org/outcome/compFull.asp.

Anderson, G. F., Hussey, P. S., Frogner, B. K., & Waters, H. R. (2005). Health spending in the United States and the rest of the world. *Health Affairs*, **24**, 903–914.

Association of American Medical Colleges. (1998). *Learning Objectives for Medical Student Education: Guidelines for Medical Schools*. Washington, DC: Author.

Barondess, J. A. (2003). Medicine and professionalism. *Archives of Internal Medicine*, **163**: 145–149.

Benson, J. A. (2002). Professionalism: Reviving or redrawing the social contract. *Annals of Allergy, Asthma & Immunology*, **89**, 114–117.

Bertram, C. (2004). *Rousseau* and the Social Contract. London: Routledge.

Bickel, J., & Brown, A. J. (2005). Generation X: Implications for faculty recruitment and development in academic health centers. *Academic Medicine*, **80**, 205–210.

Blackburn, S. (1996). *Oxford Dictionary of Philosophy*. Oxford: Oxford University Press.

Blendon, R. J., Schoen, C., Donelan, K., et al. (2001). Physicians views on quality of care: A five country comparison. *Health Affairs*, **20**, 233–243.

Bloche, M. G. (1999). Clinical loyalties and the social purposes of medicine. *JAMA*, **281**, 268–274.

Bloom, S. W. (2002). Professionalism in the practice of medicine. *The Mount Sinai Journal of Medicine*, **69**, 398–403.

Blumenthal, D. (1994). The vital role of professionalism in health care reform. *Health Affairs,* **13**, 252–256.

Blumenthal, D. (1999). Health care reform at the close of the 20th century. *New England Journal of Medicine,* **340**, 1916–1920.

Blumenthal, D. (2000). Employer-sponsored health insurance in the United States- origins and implications. *New England Journal of Medicine,* **355**: 82–88.

British Medical Association. (2005). *Data Bank.*

British Medical Association. (2008) *Data Bank.*

Brennan, T. (2002). Physician's professional responsibility to improve the quality of care. *Academic Medicine,* **77**, 973–980.

Brewbaker, W. S. (2002). Will physician unions improve health system performance? *Journal of Health Politics, Policy, and Law,* **27**, 575–604.

Broadbent, J., & Laughlin, R. (1997). 'Accounting logic' and controlling professionals. In J. Broadbent, M. Dietrich, & J. Roberts (Eds), *The End of Professions? The Restructuring of Professional Work* (pp 34–50). London: Routledge.

Brown, P., Zavetoski, S., McCormick, S., Morello-Frosch, R., & Altman, G. (2004). Embodied health movements: new approaches to social movements in health. *Sociology of Health & Illness,* **26**, 50–80.

Brownlie, J., & Howson, A. (2006). 'Between the demands of truth and government': Health practitioners, trust and immunization work. *Social Science & Medicine,* **62**, 433–443.

Callaghan, G., & Wistow, G. (2006). Governance and public involvement in the British National Health Service: understanding difficulties and developments. *Social Science & Medicine,* **63**, 2289–2300.

Canadian Medical Association. (2005). *Office of Members, Divisions, and Affiliates.* Data Bank.

Carr-Saunders, A. M., & Wilson, P. A. (1933). *The Professions.* Oxford: Clarendon Press.

Castonguay, C. (1976). The future of self-regulation. The view from Quebec. In P. Slayton., & M. Trebilcock (Eds), *The Professions and Public Policy* (pp. 61–71). Toronto,: University of Toronto Press.

Coburn, D. Professional powers in decline: Medicine in a changing Canada. (1993) In "The changing medical profession: An international perspective." Hafferty F. W., McKinlay J. B. (Eds) Oxford University Press; New York: pp. 92–104.

Cohen, J. (2000). White coats should not have union labels. *New England Journal of Medicine,* **342**, 431–434.

Cohen, J. J., Cruess, S. R. Davidson, C. (2007). Alliance between society and medicine: the public's stake in medical professionalism. JAMA. 298: 670–673.

Coulahan, J. (2005). Today's professionalism: engaging the mind but not the heart. *Academic Medicine,* **80**, 892–898.

Crocker, L. G. (1968). *Rousseau's Social Contract: An Interpretive Essay.* Cleveland: Case Western Reserve University Press.

Cruess, R. L. (1993). Locke, Rousseau and the modern surgeon. *Journal of Pediatric Orthopedics,* **13**, 108–112.

Cruess R. L., & Cruess, S. R. (1997). Teaching medicine as a profession in the service of healing. *Academic Medicine,* **72**, 941–952.

Cruess, R. L., & Cruess, S. R. (2008). Expectations and obligations: professionalism and medicine's social contract with society. *Perspectives in Medicine & Biology*, **51**, 579–598.

Cruess, R. L., Cruess, S. R., & Johnston S. E. (1999). Professionalism: An ideal to be sustained. *Lancet*, **256**, 156–159.

Daniels, N. (1978). On the picket lines: Are doctor's strikes ethical? *Hastings Center Report*, **8**, 24–29.

Daniels, N. (2008). *Just Health Care*. Cambridge: Cambridge University Press.

Davies, P., & Glasspool, J. A. (2003). Patients and the new contracts. *BMJ*, **326**, 1099.

Davis, M., & Churchill, L. R. (1991). Autonomy and the common weal. *Hasting Center Report*, **21**, 25–31.

Detsky, A. S., & Naylor, C. D. (2004). Canada's health care system- reform delayed. *New England Journal of Medicine*, **349**, 804–810.

Donaldson, L. (2006). *Good Doctors, Safer Patients. Proposals to Strengthen the System to Assure and Improve the Performance of Doctors and to Protect the Safety of Patients*. London: Department of Health.

Donaldson, T., & Dunfee, T. W. (1999). *Ties That Bind in Business Ethics: A Social Contracts Approach to Business Ethics*. Cambridge, MA.: Harvard University Business School Press.

Donaldson, T., & Dunfee, T. W. (1999). Ties that bind in business ethics: Social contracts and why they matter. *Journal of Banking and Finance*, **26**, 1853–1865.

Dunning, A. J. (1999). Status of the doctor – present and future. *Lancet*, **354** (supplement), S IV 18.

Edwards, N., Kornacki, M. J., & Silversin, J. (2002). Unhappy doctors: What are the causes and what can be done? *BMJ*, **324**, 835–838.

Elliot, P. (1972). *The Sociology of the Professions*. London.: Macmillan Press.

Feldman, D. S., Novack, D. S., & Graceley, E. (1998). Effects of managed care on physician–patient relationships, quality of care, and the ethical practice of medicine. *Archives of Internal Medicine*, **158**, 1626–1633.

Ferlie, E. B., & Shortell, S. M. (2001). Improving the quality of health care in the United States and the United Kingdom: a framework for change. *Milbank Quarterly*, **79**, 281–315.

Freddi, G., & Bjorkman, J. W. (1989). *Controlling Medical Professionals: The Comparative Politics of Health Governance*. London: Sage.

Freidson, E. (1970). *Professional Dominance: The Social Structure of Medical Care*. Chicago, IL: Aldine.

Freidson, E. (2001). *Professionalism, the Third Logic*. Chicago, IL: University of Chicago Press.

Gallopin, G. C., Funtowicz, S., O'Connor, M., & Ravetz, J. (2001). Science for the twenty-first century: from social contract to the scientific core. *International Social Science Journal.*, **53**, 219–229.

General Medical Council. (2006). *Good Medical Practice*. London.

Gibbons, M. (1999). Science's new social contract with society. *Nature*, **402**, C81–C84.

Gillon, R., Higgs, R., Boyd, K., Callaghan, B., & Hoffenberg, R. (2001). Wanted: A social contract for medicine. *BMJ*, **323**, 64.

Gough, J. W. (1957). *The Social Contract: A Critical Study of Its Development*. Oxford: The Clarendon Press.

Gruen, R. L, Pearson, S. D., & Brennan, T. A. (2004). Physician-Citizens: Public roles and professional obligations. *JAMA*, **291**, 94–98.

Hafferty, F., & McKinley, J. B. (1996). *The Changing Medical Profession: An International Perspective*. Oxford: Oxford University Press.

Hafferty, F. W., & Light, D. W. (1995). Professional dynamics and the changing nature of medical work. *Journal of Health and Social Behavior*, (extra issue), 132–153.

Hall, M. A. (2005). The importance of trust for ethics, law, and public policy. *Cambridge Quarterly of Health Care Ethics*, **14**, 156–167.

Ham, C., & Alberti, K. J. (2002). The medical profession, the public, and the government. *BMJ*, **324**, 838–842.

Haug, M. (1973). Deprofessionalization: An alternate hypothesis for the future. *Sociological Review Monograph*, **20**, 195–211.

Hellinger, F. J., & Young, G. J. (2001). An analysis of physician antitrust exemption legislation: adjusting the balance of power. *JAMA*, **286**, 83–88.

Henningson, J. A. (2002). Why the numbers are dropping in general surgery: The answer no one wants to hear- lifestyle. *Archives of Surgery*, **137**, 255–256.

Iglehart, J. K. (2005). The emergence of physician-owned specialty hospitals. *New England Journal of Medicine*, **352**, 78–84.

Ihara, C. K. (1988). Collegiality as a professional virtue. In A. Flores (Ed), *Professional Ideals'* (pp. 40–46). Belmont, CA.: Wadsworth Press.

Inui, T. S. (1992). The social contract and the medical school's responsibilities. In K. L. White, & J. E. Connelly (Eds), *The Medical School's Mission and the Population's Health: Medical Education in Canada, the United Kingdom, the United States, and Australia* (pp. 23–52). New York: Springer Verlag.

Irvine, D. (1999). The performance of doctors; the new professionalism. *Lancet*, **353**, 1174–1177.

Irvine, D. (2003). *The Doctor's Tale: Professionalism and Public Trust*. Abington, UK: Radcliffe Medical Press.

Johnson, T. (1972). *Professions and Power*. London: Macmillan Press.

Jones, R. (2002). Declining altruism in medicine. *BMJ*, **324**, 624–625.

Kearney, M. (2000). *A Place of Healing: Working with Suffering in Living and Dying*. Oxford: Oxford University Press.

Kennedy, D. (1997). *Academic Duty*. Cambridge, MA: Harvard University Press.

Kirby, M. (2002). *The Health of Canadians – The Federal Role: Final Report of the Standing Senate Committee on Social Affairs, Science, and Technology*. Ottawa: Government of Canada.

Kirp, D. L. (2003). *Shakespeare, Einstein, and the Bottom Line: The Marketing of Higher Education*. Cambridge, MA: Harvard University Press.

Klein, R. (1983). *The Politics of the National Health Service*. Harlow, UK: Longmans.

Klein, R. (1990). The state and the profession: the politics of the double bed. *BMJ*, **301S**, 700–702.

Klein, R. (1995). *The New Politics of the National Health Service* (3rd ed). Harlow, UK: Longmans.

Krause, E. (1996). *Death of the Guilds: Professions, States and the Advance of Capitalism, 1930 to the Present*. New Haven: Yale University Press.

Kultgen, J. (1988) *Ethics and Professionalism*. Philadelphia: University of Pennsylvania Press.

Kurlander, J. K., Morin, K., & Wynia, M. K. (2004). The social-contract model of professionalism: baby or bathwater? *American Journal of Bioethics*, **4**, 33–36.

Laugeson, M. J., & Rice, T. (2003). Is the doctor in? The evolving role of organized medicine in health policy. *Journal of Health Politics, Policy and Law*, **28**, 289–316.

Le Grand, J. (1997). Knights, knaves or pawns? Human behavior and social policy. *Journal of Social Policy*, **26**, 149–169.

Le Grand, J. (2003). *Motivation, Agency, and Public Policy: Of Knights and Knaves, Pawns and Queens*. Oxford: Oxford University Press.

Levinson, W., & Lurie, N. (2004). When most doctors are women: what lies ahead? *Annals of Internal Medicine*, **141**, 471–479.

Lewis, H. R. (2006). *Excellence without a Soul*. New York: Public Affairs.

Light, D. W. (2001). The medical profession and organizational change: From professional dominance to countervailing power. In C. E. Bird, P. Conrad, & A. M. Fremont (Eds), *Handbook of Medical Sociology* (5th ed) (pp. 201–216). Upper Saddle River, NJ: Prentice Hall.

Lubchenko, J. (1998). Entering the century of the environment: A new social contract for science. *Science*, **279**, 491–497.

Ludmerer, K. M. (1999). *Time to Heal*. Oxford: Oxford University Press.

Marchildon G. (2006). Health systems in transition: Canada. eds: Allin S. and Mossialos E. Toronto, ON. University of Toronto Press.

Masters, R. D., & Masters, J. R. (1978). *On the Social Contract* (including a new translation). New York: St. Martin's Press.

May, W. F. (1975). Code, covenant, contract, or philanthropy. *Hastings Center Report*, **5**, 29–38.

McCurdy, L., Goode, L. D., Inui, et al. (1997). Fulfilling the social contract between medical schools and the public. *Academic Medicine*, **72**, 1063–1070.

McKinley, J. B., & Arches, J. (1985). Toward the proletarianization of physicians. *International Journal of Health Services*, **15**, 161–195.

McKinley, J. B., & Marceau, L. D. (2002). The end of the golden age of doctoring. *International Journal of Health Services*, **32**, 379–416.

Mechanic, D. (1991). Sources of countervailing power in medicine. *Journal of Health Politics, Policy, and Law*, **16**, 585–498.

Mechanic, D. (2003). Physician discontent: Challenges and opportunities. *JAMA*, **290**, 941–946.

Mechanic, D. (2004). In my chosen doctor I trust. *BMJ*, **329**, 1418–1419.

Mechanic, D., & Schlesinger, M. (1996). The impact of managed care on patient's trust in medical care and their physicians. *JAMA*, **275**, 1693–1697.

Mello, M. M., Studdert, D. M., DesRoches, C. M., Peugh, R., Brennan, T., & Sage, W. (2004). Caring for patients in a malpractice crisis: Physician satisfaction and quality of care. *Health Affairs*, **23**, 42–50.

Meslin, E. M. (1987). The moral cost of the Ontario physicians' strike. *Hastings Center Report*, **17**, 11–14.

Moran, M., & Wood, B. (1993). *States, Regulation and the Medical Profession*. Buckingham, UK: Open University Press.

Morone, J. A. and Kilbreth, E. H. (2002). Power to the people? Restoring citizen participation. J Health Politics, Policy, and Law. **28**, 271–288.

Morreim, E. H. 2002. Professionalism and clinical autonomy in the practice of medicine. *The Mount Sinai Journal of Medicine,*. **69**, 370–377.

Page, S. (2004). How physicians' organizations compete: Protectionism and efficiency. *Journal of Health Politics, Policy, and Law*, **29**, 75–105.

Paris, J. J., & Post, S. G. (2000). Managed care, cost, control, and the common good. *Cambridge Quarterly Journal of Ethics*, **9**, 182–188.

Parsons, T. (1939). The Professions and Social Structure. *Social Forces*, **17**, 457–467.

Parsons, T. (1951). *The Social System*. New York: Free Press.

Pellegrino, E. D. (1990). The medical profession as a moral community. *Bulletin New York Academy of Medicine*, **66**, 221–232.

Pellegrino, E. D., & Relman, A. (1999). Professional medical associations: Ethical and practical guidelines. *JAMA*, **282**, 1954–1956.

Pescolido, B. A., McLeod, J., Alegria, M. (2000). Confronting the second social contract: the place of medical sociology in research and policy for the twenty-first century. in "Handbook of Medical Sociology", 5th edition. Eds. Bird, C. E., Conrad, P., Fremont, A. M. Upper Saddle River NJ. Prentice Hall. 411–426.

Peterson, M.A. (2003). Who shall lead? *Journal of Health Politics, Policy, and Law*, **28**, 181–194.

Pham, H. H., Devers, K. J., May, J. H., & Berenson, R. (2004). Financial pressures spur physician entrepreneurialism. *Health Affairs*, **23**, 70–82.

Rawls, J. (1999). *A Theory of Justice*. Cambridge, MA: Harvard University Press.

Rawls, J. (2003). *Justice as Fairness: A Restatement*. Cambridge, MA: Harvard University Press.

Rayack, E. Professional Power and American Medicine. (1967). *The Economics of the American Medical Association*. Cleveland: World.

Rettig, R. A. (1996). The social contract and the treatment of kidney failure. *JAMA*, **275**, 1123–1126.

Romonow, R. (2002). Report of the Royal Commission on the Future of Health Care in Canada. Ottawa, ON: Government of Canada.

Rosen, R., & Dewar, S. (2004). *On Being a Good Doctor: Redefining Medical Professionalism for Better Patient Care*. London: King's Fund.

Rosenbaum, S. (2003). The impact of United States law on medicine as a profession. *JAMA*, **289**, 1546–1166.

Rosenbaum S., Frankford, D. M., Moore, B., & Borzi, P. (1999). Who should determine when health care is medically necessary. *New England Journal of Medicine*, **340**, 229–232.

Rosenblatt, R. E., Shaw, S., & Rosenbaum, S. (1997). *Law and the American Health Care System*. New York: Foundation Press.

Royal College of Physicians and Surgeons of Canada. CanMEDS. (2000). Project. Skills for the New Millennium: Report of the Societal Needs Working Group. Retrieved 2 July 2010 from: http://rcpsc.medical.org.canmeds/CanMEDS e.pdf.

Royal College of Physicians of London. (2005). *Doctors in Society: Medical Professionalism in a Changing World*. London: Author.

Salter, B. (2001). Who rules? The new politics of medical regulation. *Social Science and Medicine*, **52**, 871–883.

Salter, B. (2003). Patients and doctors: reformulating the UK health policy community? *Social Science and Medicine*, **57**, 927–936.

Samanta, A., & Samanta, J. (2004). Regulation of the medical profession: fantasy, reality, and legality. *Journal of Royal Society of Medicine*, **97**, 211–218.

Schlesinger, M. A. (2002). Loss of faith: The sources of reduced political legitimacy for the American medical profession. *Milbank Quarterly*, **80**, 185–235.

Schoen, C., Osborn, R., Huynh, P. T., et al. (2004). Primary care and health system performance: Adult's experiences in five countries. *Health Affairs*, **23**, 487–503.

Schroeder, S. A., Zones, J. S., & Showstack, J. A. (1989). Academic medicine as a public trust. *JAMA*, **262**, 803–812.

Secretary of State for Health. (2007). *Trust, Assurance, and Safety – The Regulation of Health Professionals in the 21st Century*. London: Stationery Office.

Slaughter, S., & Rhoades, G. (2005). From 'endless frontier' to 'basic science for use': social contracts between science and society. *Science Technology and Human Values*, **30**, 536–572.

Smith, J. (2004). *Safegaurding Patients: Lessons from the Past – Proposals for the Future. Command Paper CM 6394*. London : The Shipman Inquiry. Retrieved 17 March 2005 from www.the-shipman-inquiry.org.uk/reports.asp.

Smith, R. (1993). All changed, changed utterly. British medicine will be transformed by the Bristol case. *BMJ*, **316**, 1917–1918.

Smith, R. J. (2001). Why are doctors so unhappy? *BMJ*, **322**, 1073–1074.

Smith, R. J. (2002). Take back your mink, take back your pearls. *BMJ*, **325**, 1047–1048.

Smith, R. J. (2004). Towards a global social contract. *BMJ*, **338**, 743.

Stacey, M. (1992). *Regulating British Medicine: The General Medical Council*. Chichester, UK.: John Wiley and Sons.

Stevens, R. (1996). *Medical Practice in Modern England: The Impact of Specialization and State Medicine*. New Haven: Yale University Press.

Stevens, R. (2001). Public roles for the medical profession in the United States: Beyond theories of decline and fall. *Milbank Quarterly*, **79**, 327–353.

Stevens, R. (2002). Themes in the history of medical professionalism. *The Mount Sinai Journal of Medicine*, **69**, 357–362.

Studdert, D. M., Mello, M. M., & Brennan T. (2004). Medical malpractice. *New England Journal of Medicine*, **350**, 283–292.

Sullivan, W. (1999). What is left of professionalism after managed care. *Hastings Center Report*, **29**, 7–13.

Sullivan, W. (2005). *Work and Integrity: The Crisis and Promise of Professionalism in North America* (2nd. Ed). San Francisco, CA: Jossey-Bass.

Starr, P. (1982). *The Social Transformation of American Medicine*. New York: Basic Books.

Starr, P. (1984). *The Social Transformation of American Medicine*. New York: Basic Books.

Swick, H. (2000). Towards a normative definition of professionalism. *Academic Medicine*, **75**, 612–616.

Swick, H. M, Bryan, C. W., Longo, L. D., (2006). Beyond the Charter: reflections on medical professionalism. Perspectives in Med and Biol, 49: 263–275.

Torrance, G. M. (1987). Socio-historical overview. In G. M. Torrance, & D. Coburn (Eds), *Health and Canadian Society – Sociological Perspectives* (pp. 6–33). Markham, ON: Fitzhenry and Whitesides.

Touhy, C. H. (1999). Dynamics of a changing health sphere: The United States, Britain, and Canada. *Health Affairs*, **18**, 114–134.

Tuohy, C. H. (2003). Agency, contract, and governance: Shifting shapes of accountability in the health care arena. *Journal of Health Politics, Policy and Law*, **29**, 195–215.

Vaughan, P. (1975). *Doctors Commons. A Short History of the British Medical Association.* London: Heineman.

Vogel, D. (1986). *National Styles of Self-Regulation*. Ithaca, NY: Cornell University Press.

Wells, A. W. (2004). Reevaluating the social contract in American medicine. *Virtual Mentor*, **6**, Retrieved 2 July 2010 from http://www.ama-assn.org/ama/pub/category/12199.html.

Williams-Jones, B., & Burgess, M. (2004). Social contract theory and just decision making: lessons from genetic testing for the BRCA mutations. *Kennedy Institute of Ethics Journal*, **14**, 115–1142.

Wolf, S. M. (1994). Health care reform and the future of physician ethics. *Hastings Center Report*, **24**, 28–41.

Wolinsky, H., & Brune, T. (1994). *The Serpent on the Staff: The Unhealthy Politics of the American Medical Association.* New York: G P Putnam's Sons.

World Medical Association. (2005). *Medical Ethics Manual.* Ferney-Voltaire Cedex, France: World Medical Association.

Wynia, M. K., Latham, S. R., Kao, A. C., Berg, J., & Emanuel, L. L. (1999). Medical professionalism in society. *New England Journal of Medicine*, **314**, 1612–1616.

Zuger, A. (2004). Dissatisfaction with medical practice. *New England Journal of Medicine*, **350**, 69–75.

Chapter 11

The role of psychiatrists and their professional associations in the regulation and performance management of mental health services

Paul Lelliott

Introduction

As doctors, psychiatrists are subject to a range of regulatory and developmental activities to assure the quality of their individual medical practice. At the core is medical regulation whose purpose is to detect and to impose sanctions on those whose practice falls below minimum standards. Systems for re-licensing and recertification might go further than the detection of outliers and require that a psychiatrist demonstrates the quality of his or her individual practice as shown by, for example, the results of clinical audit or the views of colleagues and patients elicited through multi-source feedback. There might also be a requirement that a psychiatrist proves his or her commitment to personal development by participating in educational activities. Those who work in managed organizations might be subject to supervision and appraisal. Professional associations contribute to the process of assuring quality of practice of individual doctors by setting educational standards for doctors in training, backed by examinations that control membership, and by encouraging and supporting ongoing professional development.

All of these activities aimed at maintaining standards of medical practice are necessary to ensure that high-quality care is provided for patients. However, they are not sufficient on their own. This is particularly true in a specialty such as mental health care where doctors often work as members of multidisciplinary teams and sometimes within large provider organizations. It is quite possible for a psychiatrist who has never come to the attention of a medical regulator, who has met all educational requirements, and who participates actively in ongoing professional development to be part of a team or of a larger organization that provides poor quality care to patients.

Individual doctors have a responsibility to identify organizational problems that adversely affect the quality of care and to bring these to the attention of those within their employing organization with the authority to rectify the problem. However, they often have limited power to ensure that necessary changes are made. At the regional and national levels, the external levers for regulation and performance management of health care services that are ultimately responsible for assuring the quality of care, are often separate from those that regulate and manage the performance of individual doctors.

The provision of high-quality mental health care requires both professional regulation of the clinicians providing that care and regulation and performance management of the services that employ those clinicians. This chapter presents a brief overview of the challenge of improving quality of health care and argues that psychiatrists and their professional bodies should participate more actively in quality improvement activities beyond the narrow confines of assuring the quality of medical practice. The potential for wider engagement with the regulation and performance management of services is illustrated by describing quality improvement work undertaken by the Royal College of Psychiatrists and how this relates to the national system that regulates health care in England.

The health care quality challenge

Quality has come to the forefront of health care policy in many countries. This is certainly true for those countries in Western Europe that are long-standing members of the European Union (Legido-Quigley, McKee, Nolte, & Glinos, 2008) and for the United States (Institute of Medicine, 2001). The main driver has been increased recognition of the wide variation in quality of health care both between countries and between services within countries (Institute of Medicine, 2001; Organization for Economic Co-operation and Development, 2007; The Commonwealth Fund, 2006) coupled with concern about the benefit to the population of increased spending on health care over the past decade. As far as the latter is concerned, there is little evidence that in the developed world there is a clear association between level of funding of health care and its quality (Fisher, Goodman, Skinner, & Bonner, 2009).

Most commentators include a range of dimensions in their definition of quality including effectiveness, efficiency, access, safety, equity, appropriateness, timeliness, acceptability, patient-centredness, and patient satisfaction. Factors that adversely affect these dimensions of quality operate at a number of levels (Donabedian, 1988). At the core is the interaction between a clinician and the patient. Quality at this level depends on the clinician possessing both technical proficiency, which requires knowledge and judgement, and the ability to manage interpersonal relationships. The latter, which is particularly important in the practice of psychiatry, enables the patient to communicate the information necessary for a diagnosis to be made as well as their preferences for treatment, and equips the clinician to inform and motivate the patient to collaborate with the agreed care plan.

The second level at which factors that influence quality operate is the context within which care is provided. In mental health care, in addition to the physical environment of the inpatient or community setting where care is provided, it includes the availability of workers from the other disciplines essential for high-quality care, integrated information systems, and good communication links between different elements of service and between secondary and primary care. The context also includes the extent to which administrative support is effective in ensuring efficient care processes and whether those who manage teams and services possess the leadership skills required to get the best from staff.

The third level, which is essential to the implementation of care, takes account of the patient and their families and carers who have their perspective on quality and who must take some responsibility for it.

The fourth level is the wider community. This influences access to care and therefore quality issues relating to equity. In mental health care access is influenced by factors such as levels of social deprivation and the ethnic composition of the local population. Other factors at this level are the political and societal forces that, for example, influence attitudes to mental illness and resulting stigma and discrimination against people with mental health problems and against the services and clinicians who provide care. These factors also influence the level of priority that mental health and mental health care services are given by national health care systems and by government.

The levers for improving the quality of health care

Although national health care systems vary greatly along a number of dimensions – publicly versus privately managed, centralized versus devolved authority, priorities set by governments versus determined by market forces, managerialism versus clinically led – most have a common set of interconnected levers that can be applied to affect the quality of health care. These can be broadly defined as follows:

1 *Policy guidance and directives* from regional or national government. These might include the setting of national targets or objectives in areas of health care that are considered national or regional priorities.

2 *Standard setting.* Broadly, standards fall into two categories: those that define high-quality clinical practice and those that define high quality in the organization and delivery of care.

3 *Regulation of services.* This might include a requirement that services register, or are 'certified'. This entails an organization demonstrating that it meets the minimum essential and common quality standards that are considered necessary to be permitted to provide health care services to the public at all.

4 *Performance management.* At the national or regional level this might be undertaken by the same external body that regulates or registers services. Performance management sets a level or a series of levels of performance that should be above the basic, minimal level required for registration. There are usually a set of predetermined sanctions for failure to pass the threshold and, sometimes, rewards for exceeding it.

5 *Public reporting of performance of provider services.* This reporting can either be local, for example, as part of an annual report by a provider service to the local population and/or local health care community, or national through, for example, national league tables of performance against such measures as clinical outcomes, care processes – such as waiting times – or patient experience as elicited through patient surveys.

6 *Contracts for services or items of care* often describe and commit health care providers parties to an agreed level of performance. If the provider fails to achieve this, the commissioner will not pay in full for the services offered to the patients for whom it has made the contract. In the same way that poor performance might result in financial penalties, performance that exceeds the contracted level may be rewarded through incentives. Ultimately, failure to meet the contracted level of quality might result in the services being contracted for elsewhere.

7 *Management boards* should be ultimately accountable for the quality of care provided by their provider organization and should set their own objectives and goals for the quality of care provided. They are responsible for ensuring that they give as much attention to clinical governance as they do to financial governance.

8 *Peer review and accreditation.* A national or regional regulator may use inspection visits by review teams to evaluate or investigate quality and the term 'accreditation' might be used to describe a process that affirms that an organization meets basic minimal standards and so is fit to provide health care. In addition, in a number of countries over the past few decades,

a range of non-governmental organizations have accredited health care organizations as part of a voluntary process. Some of these accredit whole health care providers; others focus on parts of provider organizations such as clinical teams, departments, or individual hospital wards. These voluntary accreditation programmes often work above the level of assuring that minimum standards are met and encourage services to aspire for excellence and work to use the recurring and cyclical nature of the review process to promote continuing improvement over time.

The role of the profession in the regulation and performance management of services

The mission statements or stated aims of some professional associations for psychiatrists suggest that they see their role as extending beyond the narrower activities of setting clinical and educational standards for doctors to that of working to improve the overall quality of care. The first of the stated aims of the Royal College of Psychiatrists is to 'set standards and promote excellence in psychiatry and mental health care'; the Royal Australian and New Zealand College of Psychiatrists 'is committed to creating better outcomes for mental health in the community' and part of the mission of the American Psychiatric Association is 'to promote the highest-quality care for individuals with mental disorders (including mental retardation and substance-related disorders) and their families'.

Despite these broad aims, a review of quality assurance systems in the European Union suggested that the work of professional associations is more focused on influencing the behaviour and enhancing the standing of the doctors who are their members. This review concluded that 'in general, [professional] associations work in three broad areas: negotiating on behalf of their members, tackling unprofessional behaviour and actively enhancing professional standards' (Legido-Quigley et al., 2008; p. 191).

Professional associations and their members can only achieve the broader aim of improving the quality of mental health care and of the outcomes for patients if they engage actively with all of the levers that influence quality and at all levels of the health care system. The rest of this chapter describes the potential role that psychiatrists and their professional associations might play in the wider field of regulation and performance management of mental health services and illustrates this with examples drawn from the work of the Royal College of Psychiatrists. First it is necessary to briefly describe how health care regulation and performance management operate in England.

Regulation and performance management of health care in England

With the delegation of political control and budgets to devolved national governments, the health care services of the four countries that comprise the United Kingdom have diverged. This has included divergence in the central mechanisms for assuring quality (Alvarez-Rosete, Bevan, Mays, & Dixon, 2005). In England the emphasis has been on national targets, market-style incentives, and external regulation.

Before 1999, there were no formal structures for regulation and performance management of health care services in England, including mental health, and little by way of systematic assurance of the quality of clinical care or of the clinical services that delivered this care. The performance management system has been transformed since then. From 2000 implementation of mental health care policy in England was driven by the National Service Framework for Mental Health (Department of Health, 1999) and the NHS Plan (Department of Health, 2000). The former defined the components of a good mental health service and the latter announced additional investment and set targets for mental health providers. Performance against these targets was monitored by a regime of self-assessment and external inspection by the Commission for Health Improvement and its successor body the Health Care Commission. In 2004, a second and independent regulator, Monitor, became involved in performance managing those NHS provider organizations that successfully applied to become 'foundation trusts' and so earned a greater degree of freedom from central government. Standards for clinical practice in England are set by the National Institute for Health and Clinical Excellence (NICE), whose first ever clinical practice guideline, published in 2002, was on a mental health topic – schizophrenia.

From 2010, the performance management system for health care services in England was strengthened further. The Care Quality Commission (CQC), which subsumed the Health Care Commission, is now the national inspectorate for health care services in England. From April 2010, and for the first time, all mental health care providers are required to register with the CQC that has powers to suspend, cancel, or impose conditions on registration, issue warnings and penalty notices, or prosecute provider organizations. Monitor continues to also play a role in performance managing the increasing number of mental health provider services that have become foundation trusts – about one-half of mental health services were foundation trusts by the summer of 2009.

At the same time as the regulators had been granted new powers, a new policy direction for the NHS was announced that increases the reach of regulation into the area of clinical practice and is likely to require clinicians to be more active participants in the performance management of the health care services that employ them. The NHS *Next Stage Review* (Department of Health, 2008), which was written by Lord Darzi a government minister, who was also a practicing surgeon, places clinical quality at the centre of the NHS and envisages a much stronger leadership role for clinicians in developing local services. Darzi proposes a number of measures to achieve this vision:

- The development by NICE of 'quality standards' that are defined as 'a set of specific, concise statements acting as markers of high-quality, cost-effective care across a pathway or a clinical area. NICE quality standards are derived from the best available evidence' (National Institute for Health and Clinical Excellence, 2009). These quality standards go beyond recommendations for clinical decisions by individual practitioners to describe the care structures and processes required to deliver high-quality care with regard to clinical effectiveness, patient safety, and patient experience.
- The development of a set of quality indicators or 'national metrics' that enable measurement of key aspects of quality.

Table 11.1 The service accreditation and quality improvement programmes managed by the Royal College of Psychiatrists, the date they were established and the number of services participating

	Start date	Number of participants in July 2009
Service accreditation programmes		
Electroconvulsive therapy clinics	2003	108 clinics
Acute working age adult wards	2006	144 wards
Older people wards	2008	54 wards
Inpatient learning disability units	2008	42 units
Memory services	2009	34 services
Psychiatric liaison services	2009	18 teams
Service quality improvement networks		
Child and adolescent inpatient units	2001	93 units
Therapeutic communities	2002	88 communities
Child and adolescent community services	2005	80 teams
Children's learning disability services	2005	12 teams
Forensic mental health services	2006	64 services
Perinatal mental health inpatient units	2007	13 services
The prescribing observatory for mental health	2005	48 trusts

- April 2010 onwards, a requirement in law that all NHS providers publish 'quality accounts' that report to the public on the quality of services they provide in terms of safety, patient experience, and outcomes. It is intended that this information will also be made available on the NHS Choices website.
- Alterations to the commissioning and contracting system so that payments for services reflect clinical quality.
- The establishment of a 'quality observatory' by each regional strategic health authority to enable local benchmarking, development of metrics, and identification of opportunities to help frontline staff innovate and improve.

The quality improvement activities of the Royal College of Psychiatrists

Over the same period that the new regulatory framework has been put in place, the Royal College of Psychiatrists has established a programme of work intended to support improvement in the quality of mental health services in the United Kingdom. This includes national, standards-based quality improvement networks that increasingly cover the elements comprising a comprehensive mental health care system. Some of these accredit the services that take part (see Table 11.1).

The longer established networks involve a substantial proportion of all eligible services in England. For example, about 90% of all eligible units participate in the Quality Improvement Network for Inpatient Child and Adolescent Mental Health Services and more than two-thirds of all electro-convulsive therapy (ECT) clinics are members of the College's ECT Accreditation Service.

The accreditation programmes and quality improvement networks apply a set of common principles. They attempt to

- foster local ownership and trust by ensuring that the process is owned by front-line staff and incorporates true peer review;
- engage with all relevant groups including staff of all disciplines in the clinical team, senior service managers, and patients and their carers;
- be credible by ensuring that the standards are explicit, are based on best evidence, and are recognized by all relevant professional associations and that the process by which services are evaluated is transparent;
- be responsive by providing prompt feedback to participating services that includes advice and support about how to meet standards and by encouraging networking through newsletters and an email discussion group;

- focus on development: although the process of review is rigorous, and the feedback honest, the purpose of the process is to support and help units to improve in line with the standards;
- promote excellence and year-to-year improvement: participating services are encouraged to work towards achieving the highest category of accreditation 'excellence', and the standards become more difficult to attain each year as they are slowly revised upwards.

The standards that underpin the quality improvement networks and accreditation programmes cover much more than the behaviour of psychiatrists or interaction between clinicians and patients. Typically they also consider the following:
- the physical environment and facilities of the unit or team base;
- staffing, including leadership, training, and supervision;
- access, admission, and discharge;
- care and treatment processes;
- factors that relate to security and to patient and staff safety;
- (for inpatient services) 'the patient day' and access to therapies;
- links with other elements of health and social care services that work with the same patient group;
- patient rights and safeguards, including the use of the Mental Health Act.

The standards are drawn from authoritative sources to ensure that services are evaluated against accepted best practice. These include national policy documents; national guidance on policy implementation; national clinical practice guidance and standards set by national regulators; recommendations made by professional associations or by national patient organizations; and the findings of inquiries into adverse events.

The draft standards are refined, and gaps filled, by a process of consultation that takes full account of the views of frontline staff and also those of patients and their carers. They are then subject to annual review. The complete set of standards is aspirational; no service could be expected to meet every one. Standards might be categorized into (1) those that are essential to safety and good basic care, and so should be met by every service; (2) those that are indicators that a good service should meet; and (3) those that, if met, denote an excellent service. The process of selecting and categorizing standards recognizes that services are diverse and that there are different structures and configurations of service that can meet the standards.

The service standards are reviewed annually in the light of new policy and practice developments and feedback from the reviews.

The review process

Stage 1: Simple audit tools are developed and tested to support evaluation against the standards.

Stage 2: After an induction event, services undertake self-review using a range of methods.

Stage 3: The service hosts a peer-review visit by a multi-professional team that includes patients when possible.

Stage 4: A written local report is sent to the service. This includes a statement about performance against the standards, highlights achievements and issues that need attention, and gives advice and comments from the review team.

Stage 5: Action planning and implementation of findings. This is supported centrally and through the encouragement of networking between participating units by use of annual forums, newsletters, and email discussion groups.

Reviews happen on a cyclical basis (Figure 11.1), and it is expected that services demonstrate engagement in an ongoing process of improvement, working on areas that had been highlighted during the previous review.

How this activity does and could relate to service regulation and performance management

For professionally led quality improvement programmes to have the maximum impact they must work with and interact with the national and regional levers that affect the quality of health care as described above. In this section I

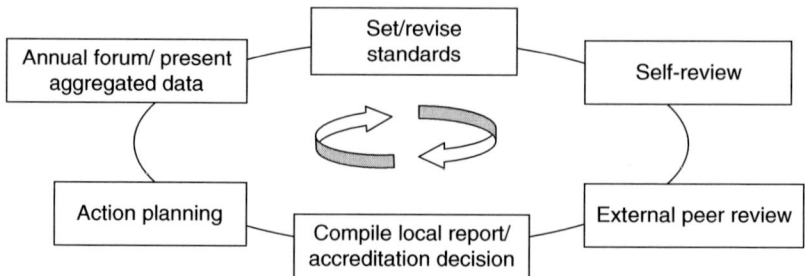

Fig. 11.1 The cyclical review process for quality improvement/accreditation programmes

describe ways in which this might happen and illustrate it with actual examples.

Promoting uptake of national policy. National guidance and directives are one source of standards for the quality improvement and accreditation programmes managed by the Royal College of Psychiatrists. There are mutual benefits in this. For the government and national health care regulators, incorporation of guidance into standards used in professionally led peer review promotes the policy position in that area of health care. For the professional association it creates an incentive for management boards of health care organizations to participate in their quality improvement programmes because they are a means of demonstrating their commitment to implementing national policy.

Supporting the implementation of standards. The Royal College of Psychiatrists' quality improvement networks are a vehicle for implementing both clinical standards, of the type contained in clinical practice guidelines, and the more organizationally oriented standards such as the new NICE 'quality standards'. The College has an active role in developing these standards through its management, in partnership with the British Psychological Society, of the NICE-funded National Collaborating Centre for Mental Health.

Where relevant, the standards that underpin the quality improvement programmes have also been 'mapped onto' other sets of standards used in regulatory activities such as the 'Core Standards for Better Health' that underpinned the 'Annual Health Check' of provider organizations by the Healthcare Commission and by its successor the Care Quality Commission (Healthcare Commission, 2009) and the risk management standards used by the NHS Litigation Authority to assess health care organizations (NHS Litigation Authority, 2009).

Regulation and performance management of services. At present the relationship between the quality improvement programmes managed by the College and the work of the English health care regulators is poorly defined. Although there have been occasions when the Care Quality Commission has used information derived from the College programmes, for example, a review of inpatient services by the Healthcare Commission of inpatient units took account of the accreditation status of the wards' ECT clinics (Healthcare Commission, 2008), these have been the exception and not the rule. There are obvious benefits for all parties from closer collaboration between the regulator and those managing professionally led quality improvement programmes (Lelliott, 2009). These include improved quality of the data, engagement by clinicians, and the provision of a more rounded picture of the quality of the large and complex organizations that are the mainstay of some modern mental health care systems.

Regulators require high-quality and complete information about the quality of the process of clinical care, the outcomes achieved, and the level of patient satisfaction. Quality improvement networks and accreditation programmes could be an important source of this because the information is collected by, or its collection is overseen by, frontline clinicians who have an interest in its accuracy and completeness. In turn, the use of the information by regulators would legitimize and formalize the professionally led quality improvement programmes and could trigger a virtuous cycle that promotes participation and further improves the quality of data collected. For health care provider organizations, closer collaboration would reduce the risk of duplication and help them to increase positive engagement in the regulatory process by local clinicians.

Secondary mental health care for England's 50 Million people is provided by just 60 NHS mental health care providers. These are therefore large and complex organizations, that provide care from many, dispersed community and hospital settings and often across large geographical areas. Regulation which, as in England, is applied at the level of the whole provider organization cannot take account of this complexity and diversity. It is highly likely that organizations that are judged to be excellent by the regulator have elements of service that are of poor quality and vice versa. Professionally led quality improvement networks measure quality at a lower level of a health care provider organization; and often at a level that is more meaningful to clinicians and patients. This can therefore paint a more detailed picture of what is good and what could be improved.

Public reporting of performance. The detailed and accurate data that can be collected by professional associations working through clinicians can provide exactly the type of information that, if put into the public domain, will give patients and the wider public a better understanding of the quality of their local health care service and, ultimately, the ability to better exercise choice. Figures 11.2 and 11.3 draw on two of the Royal College of Psychiatrists' quality improvement programmes to illustrate the type of data that might be reported publicly. Figure 11.2 shows the wide variation between 32 anonymous mental healthcare provider organizations in the proportion of psychiatric inpatients prescribed doses of antipsychotic drugs that are above the limits recommended by the British National Formulary. This practice contravenes the recommendations of the NICE clinical practice guideline for schizophrenia. Figure 11.3 shows how 32 unnamed ECT clinics have improved, as measured by their compliance with key standards, during the first three years of their participation in the ECT Accreditation Service.

THE QUALITY IMPROVEMENT ACTIVITIES OF THE ROYAL COLLEGE OF PSYCHIATRISTS | 159

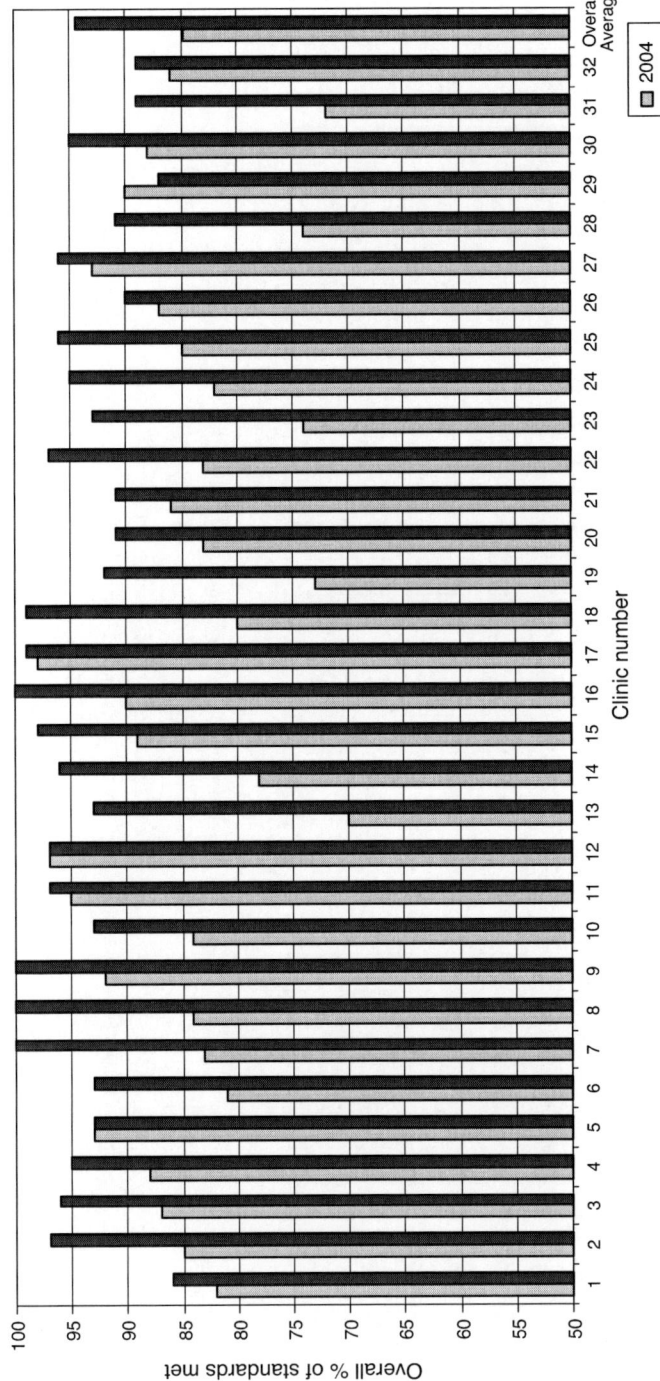

Fig. 11.2 The percentage of standards met in 2004 and 2007 by the first 32 electro-convulsive therapy (ECT) clinics to complete two full cycles of the ECT accreditation process. The information in this figure is drawn from the work of the ECT Accreditation Service.

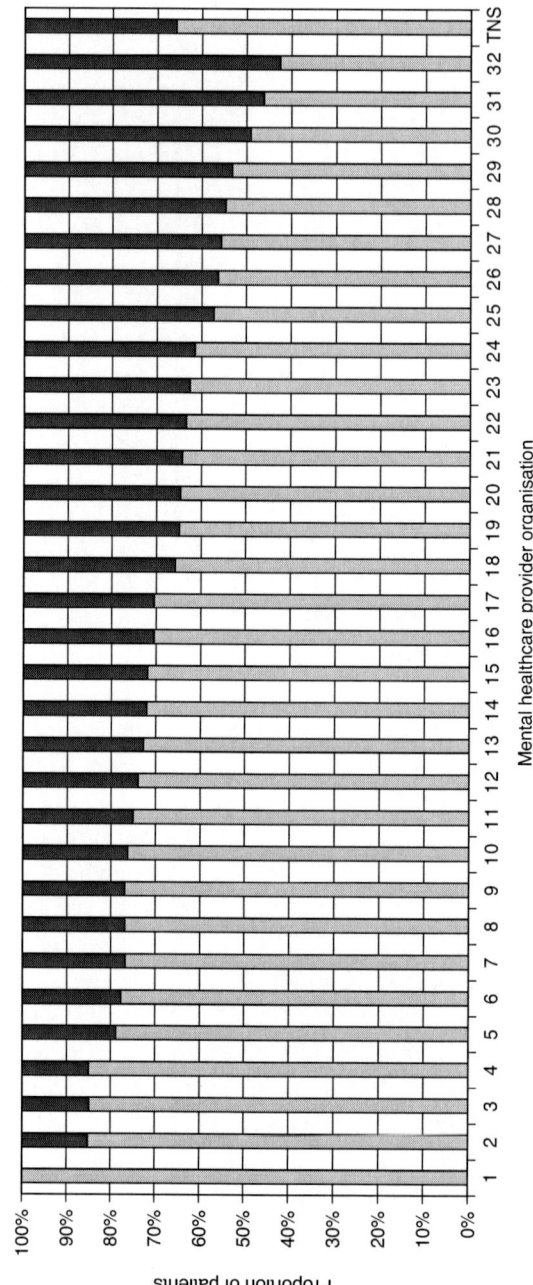

Fig. 11.3 The proportion of patients in 32 UK mental health providers who were prescribed doses of antipsychotic drugs higher than those recommended by the British National Formulary (BNF). The information in this figure is drawn from the work of the Prescribing Observatory for Mental Health. TNS = mean of the total national sample

Figures 11.2 and 11.3 illustrate a dilemma for psychiatrists and their professional associations. On the one hand, there is a powerful argument in favour of full disclosure in that doctors have a responsibility to be open and transparent and patients and the public have a right to know. On the other hand, the clinicians who participated in these quality improvement projects did so in the knowledge that the principal purpose was for them to learn about their practice and their service with the intention of then taking action to address deficits in quality. This assurance of confidentiality almost certainly increased the number of clinicians who were willing to participate and the honesty with which they laid their practice open to scrutiny by their peers. This dilemma must be overcome if professionally led quality improvement is to maximize its impact and complement service regulation (Lelliott, 2009).

Contracting and commissioning. The reports about local services generated by the quality improvement and accreditation cycle are often shared with commissioners as evidence of compliance with standards. The English national specialist commissioning group has gone a step further by making a contractual requirement that all NHS-funded medium secure units in England, both NHS-managed units and those managed by the independent sector, participate in the Quality Network for Forensic Mental Health Services.

Management boards. Most of the funding for the quality improvement networks and accreditation programmes listed in Table 11.1 comes from fees paid by provider organizations. However, because these are large organizations, and because the programmes focus on particular teams or service elements, the senior executives of these mental health care providers are not always aware of the extent of participation by their clinical staff. There is potential for boards to make greater use of the data generated by this work to assure good clinical governance and for upward reporting, including through quality accounts.

Conclusion

If psychiatrists are to optimize the health gain for their patients and professional associations are to achieve their broader goal of promoting excellence in mental healthcare, they must engage actively and constructively with the levers for national regulation and performance management of health care services. The benefits for regulators include the potential to extend their performance management activities into aspects of service delivery that are more meaningful in terms of patient outcomes and experience. However, there are risks to this closer engagement and clear rules of engagement should be negotiated that ensure that the relationship is equal and reciprocal.

References

Alvarez-Rosete, A., Bevan, G., Mays, N., & Dixon, J. (2005). Information in practice: Effect of diverging policy across the NHS. *British Medical Journal*, **331**, 946–950.

Department of Health. (1999). *National Service Framework for Mental Health: Modern Standards and Service Models*. London: Author.

Department of Health (2000). *The NHS Plan: A Plan for Investment a Plan for Reform*. London: Author.

Department of Health. (2008). High Quality Care for All: NHS Next Stage Review Final Report. London: Author.

Donabedian, A. (1988). The quality of care: How can it be assessed? *Journal of the American Medical Association*, **260**, 1743–1748.

Fisher, E., Goodman, D., Skinner, J., & Bonner, K. (2009). Health Care Spending, Quality and Outcomes: More Isn't Always Better. The Dartmouth Institute. Retrieved October 2009 from http://www.dartmouthatlas.org/atlases/Spending_Brief_022709.pdf.

Healthcare Commission. (2008). *The Pathway to Recovery: A Review of NHS Acute Inpatient Mental Health Services*. London: Author. Retrieved October 2009 from http://www.cqc.org.uk/publications.cfm?fde_id=806.

Healthcare Commission. (2009). *Criteria for Assessing Core Standards 2008/09: Mental Health and Learning Disability Trusts*. London: Author. Retrieved October 2009 from http://www.cqc.org.uk/_db/_documents/Criteria_for_assessing_core_standards_08-09_for_MHLD_trusts_200903194404.pdf.

Institute of Medicine. (2001). *Crossing the Quality Chasm: A New Health System for the 21st Century*. Washington DC: National Academy Press.

Legido-Quigley, H., McKee, M., Nolte, E., & Glinos I. A. (2008). *Assuring the Quality of Health Care in the European Union: A Case for Action*. Copenhagen: World Health Organization Regional Office.

Lelliott, P. (2009). The role of the clinical professions in the regulation of healthcare in England: Walking the tightrope. *Psychiatric Bulletin*, **33**, 321–324.

National Institute for Health and Clinical Excellence. (2009). NICE Quality Standards. Retrieved October 2009 from http://www.nice.org.uk/aboutnice/qualitystandards/qualitystandards.jsp.

NHS Litigation Authority. (2009). NHSLA Risk Management Standards for Mental Health & Learning Disability Trusts 2009/10. NHSLA. Retrieved October 2009 from http://www.nhsla.com/NR/rdonlyres/1E1FC8D6-2DFF-44D7-8AA8-B6839837B4CC/0/NHSLARMStandardsforMHLDTrusts.doc.

Organisation for Economic Co-operation and Development. (2007). *Health at a Glance: OECD Indicators*. Paris: OECD Publishing.

The Commonwealth Fund (2006). Why Not the Best? Results from a National Scorecard on U.S. Health System Performance. New York: The Commonwealth Fund.

Chapter 12

Professionalism, regulation, scrutiny, and litigation

Carole Kaplan

Introduction

The interrelationship between professionalism, regulation, scrutiny, and litigation is a highly complex one that arouses strong feeling. There is a long-held assumption that if someone behaves professionally, they probably do not need regulation, and if they do, they can certainly do it within their own professional group. Anything more formal than peer appraisal, such as formal scrutiny, has not been fully accepted and the idea of litigation has been held to be apocryphal by some.

It is important to start with definitions of the words we use. In particular, the definition of professionalism has given rise to much discussion and debate. In this chapter I will use the definition provided by the Royal College of Physicians (2005): 'Medical professionalism signifies a set of values, behaviours and relationships that underpins the trust the public has in doctors.'

Regulation can be considered as 'controlling or directing through the process of rulemaking and adjudication, or a governmental order having the force of law, or more generally control through a formalised process' (*OED*, short version). Allied to regulation are the processes of scrutiny (a careful examination or enquiry); monitoring (which gives warning so that a mistake can be avoided); and litigation (which is a context authorized by law in a court for the purpose of enforcing a right). The manner in which these different mechanisms and structures interact to enhance, or even diminish, professionalism will be explored.

Is there a reason for concern?

It has been suggested that the so-called 'scandalous' cases of Bristol, Shipman, Ledward, and others are the explanations for the impetus to regulate the medical profession. Criticism of the General Medical Council (GMC) has also served to highlight this. However, we do have to consider that there may be additional reasons that add to the call for different ways of regulation.

In 2006/2007, 5426 claims of clinical negligence were received by the NHS Litigation Authority (NHSLA). An amount of £579.3 million was paid out in connection with clinical negligence claims in the same year. The NHSLA estimates that its total liability is £9.09 billion for clinical claims. It should be noted that only 48 mental health trusts out of 59 have achieved Level 1 of the Clinical Negligence Scheme for Trusts (CNST) and only 10 have achieved Level 2. This is far below the level of acute hospitals and other NHS trusts.

Examination of the number of clinical negligence claims places those related to mental health in the top 10 of all specialties in successive years. Thus, the idea that mental health is a rare player in this area is to be challenged. The reasons (or causation) of the claims are varied but all relate to a patient and/or their families having a negative perception of the health care they have received.

In addition to this, the number of 'fitness to practice' hearings at the General Medical Council is about 300 per annum and the number of referrals to the National Clinical Assessment Service (NCAS) is 650 to date. This should at least give us cause to consider that there is justifiable cause to reconsider issues of professionalism and regulation at this time and to question whether we have a system that is working for our patients.

Approximately 8,000 second stage requests in relation to complaints have been sent to the Health Care Commission and an article in *WHICH* (October 2007) revealed that only 1 in 6 patients who had had a 'bad' health care experience complained. The reason for this small number is said to be because the patient and/or carers felt that there was 'no point' or 'they feared that future care may be affected'. Of those who did complain, only 27% were satisfied with how the concerns were handled. Therefore, even if there is an adverse experience, there may be uncertain levels of confidence in the Health Service's ability to investigate and learn from the process. Even more worrying is the hint of concern about what reaction the patient may experience if they express dissatisfaction.

There are therefore many reasons for concern about the way the medical profession is providing service to patients.

What do the problems usually relate to?

The vast majority of patients are helped by, and benefit from, contact with their doctors. A high standard is reached by most, but not all. If we set the criterion for practice as 'Is this doctor good enough to be my doctor, my mother's doctor, my child's doctor?', I believe that the vast majority of the medical profession would be fit to perform these highly responsible roles. This is reflected by the high level of confidence and trust expressed by the public in surveys and public polls. However, we must remember that patients have a need to trust their doctors, and that this may influence the rating.

The usual area of complaint is in relation to behaviour, attitudes, and conduct of individuals. The problem seems to relate to the relatively small percentage of contacts where things go wrong. Patients use words such as 'unsympathetic', 'not listening', 'dismissive', and 'patronizing' to describe some of their interactions with their doctors. Of course this is balanced by the large number of positive attributes ascribed. However, communication and attitude do cause problems. This, of course, is in addition to those cases where serious errors have been made, usually as a result of a system not working rather than as an individual alone being at fault.

Who and what is involved?

Doctors can be considered as individuals in relation to their training, professional practice, and personal issues, and also as part of a system of health care.

Doctors as individuals

In considering doctors as individuals, the description given by the Royal College of Physicians (2005) is helpful. This states that 'medicine is a vocation, in which a doctor's knowledge, clinical skills, and judgement are put to the service of protecting and restoring human well-being'. This purpose is realized through a partnership between patient and doctor, one based on mutual respect, individual responsibility, and appropriate accountability. In their day-to-day practice, doctors are committed to integrity, compassion, altruism, continuous improvement, excellence, and working in partnership with members of the wider health care team.

These standards and ways of practising should be set as expectations right from the beginning of a career in medicine. We do need to ask questions about who is suitable to train to become a doctor:

- How should we select them?
- How should we train them?
- Who are they trained by?
- Do they model professionalism?
- Will they conduct themselves professionally?
- How do we know that they will/are maintaining proper standards?

Slowly a more formalized approach is being adopted and we now see questionnaires being given to appointments committees to ask what qualities they were looking for following an interview for a place at medical school.

Questionnaires and feedback systems now abound for us to complete in relation to trainees at the time of their selection to a training scheme and at regular stages during their training, but what about assessing the trainers?

Should we not be regularly assessing the quality of the trainers in relation to the content of what they teach, and their conduct? Issues such as the trainers' ability to communicate, their way of handling interviews with patients and examinations and the way in which they talk about patients and colleagues, for example, whether they denigrate them, should be raised. We certainly need to be careful that the people who train the doctors of the future are good models for our profession. With time we should aspire to demonstrate that this has been done in a meaningful way.

Doctors, as individual professionals, must possess the correct skills and knowledge and there should be a clear career trajectory, including a leadership trajectory. To function as a professional medical practitioner, good patient relationships are essential, as is team work and also some understanding and participation in management and research. No longer is the doctor simply valued, or indeed paid, on the basis of the medical skills alone. Other qualities are also required at a high level, some of which may have been taken for granted, or their absence tolerated, in the past.

Considering professional conduct, probity is something that is marked on our appraisal forms and is a standard required of professionals. However, it is interesting how few people are able to define this and indeed to put it into effect. If we accept the definition of probity as being 'moral excellence', and then apply this to the use of time, questions about traditional ways of working are raised. For example, are court reports being prepared during Trust time and who should pay for the time to recover from jet lag? Serious questions need to be asked in relation to private practice, the use of drug company support, the use of IT, and quite simple things like making private telephone calls. The principle of two payments for the same time of work being wrong may need a more diligent application. The spending of money and, very importantly, resources that are public property, must be evaluated as to whether this is using our skills in the way that is best for our patients. Personal conduct is judged by the professional's behaviour, their ability to exercise good judgement, and this may, in many ways, be reflected in professional reputation. However, the question of whether this is enough and whether the ultimate paymaster, the patient, is satisfied with this must be posed.

Doctors as part of a system

Doctors do not operate as individuals practicing a medical skill. They are professionals who operate within teams and within organizations. The need to be an effective member of a team is becoming increasingly important to demonstrate. Many of us will have completed appraisals using different approaches and instruments. Many of these now have the views of colleagues as an integral part of the assessment. Stress and bullying are issues that trouble the health service, and doctors can be both the source and recipient of these. The need to ensure proper conduct that respects others is surely an integral part of a professional culture.

Doctors are also used by the courts and national bodies as a source of expertise. In providing expert evidence in court, a high standard is required and issues of training, skill, and practice are rightly questioned. The initiative in relation to expert witnesses, with which this college has been actively engaged, is a good example of the need to tackle this area.

Similarly, when various members of our profession operate on national bodies and provide advice, it needs to be considered whether they are representing themselves, their profession, their college, or their Trust, and the standard to which they do this. The issue of how each appointment is made and how we ensure continuation of medical clinical service is well made here. It also needs to be remembered that appointment to a national body, court work, or private work requires that the rest of the team support professional practice in relation to patients and clinical care while these individuals are away.

Demands of management also grow apace, and management teams may also need to 'backfill' the absence of a medical manager. Doctors must operate professionally as part of a system and be willing to both support and accept support. The use of time needs to be scrutinized as carefully as the use of any other resource.

Standards for systems

Standards for systems have been set by the Health Care Commission, CNST, National Institute of Clinical Excellence (NICE), the colleges, and others. It is important that these standards should be set with full clinical advice and the issue of professionals taking part in formulating these is important. Not only is it important for professionals to provide a good standard of advice when these systems are set up, but there is indeed an obligation to take part in the elucidation and implementation of these standards. It is not acceptable to say that a professional does not agree with standards that have been set by an agreed system and therefore will not take part in them. If a national standard is set and agreed through governmental mechanisms, then it is the professional's obligation to take part in this. If there is no compliance with this, then corrective measures may have to be considered.

Is regulation needed?

In my view, there is a need for the demonstration of a high level of professionalism and a clear system to ensure that default from this standard is controlled in the best interest of the public and the profession. There is no escape from the fact that there are areas and practitioners where less than professional behaviour and care have been offered, sometimes with very serious effect. Under these circumstances the process of inquiry, learning the lessons and at times a form of reparation is needed.

Who should be the regulators?

This is a very difficult question to answer, particularly given the recent tensions associated with the work of the GMC. Professional attributes are often described as incorporating autonomy, privilege, and self-regulation. The exercise of self-regulation is fiercely guarded by professionals, arguing that they are in a unique position to make informed determinations. Unfortunately, this can often be misunderstood and if self-regulation is thought by the public to allow low standards of practice, one must question whether this is acceptable. The need for clarity and transparency must be integral to any system of regulation, whether or not by the profession itself.

The capacity to self-regulate is a privilege that must be earned and is not attached to professional bodies as of right. Privilege certainly should not encompass immunity from liability. The practice of medicine relies on patients having confidence in their doctors and in my view a robust and clear system of regulation is integral to this.

How can regulation of professionalism work?

It is possible to consider the regulation of professionalism in two parts. First, may be regulation by affirmation. This may be part of the appraisal and CPD systems. The awarding of merit awards and discretionary points is a way of affirming the excellence of professional practice by a doctor. Regulation by affirmation using a 360° appraisal is also a good example of how this can be done across several domains of functioning. These forms of regulation affirm the positive aspects of the professional behaviour of a doctor and psychiatrist.

However, there is also regulation by default and this encompasses areas such as complaints, referrals to the GMC and clinical negligence litigation and other forms of litigation. These highlight the more negative aspects of consequences of behaviour.

In my view, it is our professional duty, and indeed privilege, to support and help colleagues in difficulty. There is little doubt that this is not an area in which we excel. Medical practitioners are not good at accessing and receiving health care, particularly in the area of mental health. New initiatives such as the Practitioner Health Programme make the first step to improving the situation, but there is a long way to go.

Medical practitioners are expensive to train and psychiatrists take a lot of time and resources to reach a high level of skill. When they are unwell, or in need of support, this should be identified and provided quickly. However, if it becomes apparent that a return to work is unlikely, despite reasonable adjustments having been made, progress to a conclusion is needed in a time span not measured in years. This enables the practitioner to move to other endeavours and the health service to spend public money on providing a service.

One of the areas for criticism is the length of time it can take to identify, modify, or remove unsatisfactory practice. The process of identification is often very lengthy, investigation can span years, and attempts to remediate can be multiple, inconclusive, and lengthy. Should matters be brought to an adjudication, this takes long periods to achieve and very large amounts of money are used in these processes in terms of salaries for doctors who are on 'gardening leave' and not practising, time used by those working on the process, and in stress-related difficulties for the teams working with these situations and trying to keep the service running.

Conclusion

In considering the way forward, professionals must be accountable and responsible. They must practice following principles that are held to be paramount and operate within processes that fit these principles. This system should be proactive rather than reactive for the majority. It must be possible to bring together different forms of regulation encompassing both affirmation and default processes and to bring together, from the time of entry to the medical profession until the time of retirement, a developmental career structure which enhances and supports professional behaviour. The end result should be a trusted, responsible, and healthy workforce fully engaged in the process of regulation and interested in the outcome.

References

Department of Health. (2008). *Good Doctors, Safer Patients* . London: Author.
Department of Health. (2008). *Bearing Good Witness: Proposals for Reforming the Delivery of Medical Expert Evidence in Family Law Courts* – London: Author.
National Health Service Litigation Authority – Annual Report, 2008
Szauter, K., Williams, B., Ainsworth, M. A., Callaway, M., Bulik, R., & Camp, M. G. (2003).
Student Perceptions of the Professional Behaviour of Faculty Physicians – *Medical*

Education Online (serial online), **8**:17 available from http://www.med-ed-online.org/res00067.html

AMA Code of Medical Ethics - The Council on Ethical and Judicial Affairs (CESA) http://www.ama-assn.org/

Working Party of the Royal College of Physicians. (2005). Doctors in Society. Medical Professionalism in a Changing World – Report of a Working Party. *Clinical Medicine*, **5** (6 Suppl 1), S5–S40.

Chapter 13

Psychiatry's contract with society: a personal perspective from England

Hugh Griffiths

Introduction

The relevance and role of psychiatry have long been debated and alongside significant developments in knowledge and understanding in the twentieth century, concern over its use as an instrument of social control has been a recurring theme. Even in the seventeenth century (before the word 'psychiatry' was first used), it was said that some women were incarcerated in madhouses for being disobedient, even though they were sane (Daniel Defoe quoted in Szasz, 1976). Some views that were highly antipathetic to psychiatry continued to emerge but it was not until the 1960s that the anti-psychiatry movement gained significant prominence with charismatic leaders such as R.D. Laing and Thomas Szasz directly challenging the fundamental assumptions and practices of the profession (Laing, 1960). The central tenet of the movement was that mental illness is essentially a myth (Szasz, 1972) based on a physical concept of disease that cannot be applied to psychological disorder.

Although such a belief may be regarded as narrow and significantly flawed, followers of anti-psychiatry have represented a broad range of opinion with significant areas of disagreement and some apparent inconsistency (Gijswijt-Hofstra & Porter, 1998). More recently in England, however, 'critical psychiatry' has been established (since 1999) as a network of mental health professionals, service users, and carers who are critical of current theory and practice. In particular, they are critical of what they perceive as a biological bias in psychiatry and the involvement and claims of the pharmaceutical industry. They stress the importance of social factors such as poverty, unemployment, poor housing, stigma, and social isolation (http://www.critpsynet.freeuk.com). To many, the issue may appear to be one of emphasis. Arguably, most people who work in services have an integrated concept of mental health problems that incorporates diverse factors, but the perceived relevance of these different components may vary from person to person and from one situation to another.

Despite all this, there remains widespread recognition of the importance of doctors who are interested in mental disorders, their diagnosis and treatment, and in better understanding through painstaking research. However, the important questions being posed in the early twenty-first century are less about the need for medical expertise. They are more about the best ways for doctors to contribute in a world changing exponentially. This is true across health care but arguably it is especially true in mental health where a constellation of high-level drivers for change interact uniquely with changing policy and legislation. Much of this is beyond the profession's direct sphere of influence; for example, changes at the political level such as the Human Rights Act and European legislation, changing social expectations, and so on. However, some do require psychiatrists to influence or provide leadership, particularly in the development of new knowledge, technical advance, and consensus around best practice.

Perspective from England

Over the past 10 years in England, there have been major changes and developments in mental health provision, and for adults of working age, most of this has been driven by a policy contained within a combination of the National Service Framework (NSF; Department of Health, 1999) and the *National Health Service* (NHS) Plan (Department of Health, 2000). The National Service Framework set out a comprehensive vision for the provision of mental health care, whereas the NHS Plan specified clear service objectives to achieve that vision. The government's strategy was to reform services through extra investment, to set clear goals (targets) linked to that investment, and to modernize mental health legislation (Mental Health Act 1983, amended 2007).

Although such an approach, based primarily on 'input targets', gained a mixed reception, it nevertheless led to significant increases in funding for mental health services, which were reflected in corresponding increases in the number of staff. Between 2001/2 and 2008/9 total investment in adult mental health services increased by nearly £2 billion (about 50%) with inflation taken into account (Department of Health, 2009a) and from 1997 the numbers of consultant psychiatrists had increased by 62%, clinical psychologists by 78%, and nurses by 24%. As a result, 750 new mental health teams were set up covering crisis resolution and home treatment, early intervention in psychosis, and assertive outreach (Department of Health, 2009a). However, such increases in provision (however much they may be based on good evidence) do not automatically lead to better outcomes or experience of the treatment and care provided; much of that is also dependent on effective clinical governance including a focus on quality and safety, good education and training, and the right organizational culture. Nevertheless, they do lead to fundamental changes in the configuration of services and mean that mental health professionals of all disciplines face the need to adapt their practice. This need grew with the advent of a new era of health care provision in England heralded by system reform, the next stage review (Department of Health, 2008), and a consequent emerging focus on quality and outcomes. System reform was designed to boost the efficiency and responsiveness of NHS services. To do this, the overall objective was a move away from centrally driven targets and initiatives to a system that was designed to help the NHS to be 'self-improving' as described below. Whatever view we, as individuals or groups of professionals, take of such moves, they are likely to lead to significant shifts in our working lives and the environment in which we practice. So for us to do our best for our patients and our services, we need to understand what is going on and be prepared to recognize where we can and cannot make a difference, speak out constructively when we need to, and adapt our practice as necessary.

System reform had at its core an intention to reshape the NHS so that continuous improvement was built into it. It was also intended to provide incentives to deliver better value for money. To achieve this, there were four areas of reform that should work together:

1 *Demand-side reforms* – an emphasis on patient choice together with better information available (e.g., through the NHS Choices website) and a stronger voice for service users.
2 *Supply-side reforms* – a greater diversity of service providers (including those from the voluntary and independent sectors) and more freedom to innovate and improve services. This also includes the development of foundation trusts.
3 *Transactional reforms* – developments such as standard contracts and payment by results. The intention to reward innovation and efficiency.
4 *System management reforms* – such as the development of improved regulation and agreed guidelines.

Such changes as these (and those in the current Government's plans) will lead to a system of health care that is fundamentally different from the one we have known. The central role of the NHS becomes commissioning, planning, and paying for services delivered by a variety of organizations, many of them being trusts but an increasing number that are not. Given that much mental health care is already provided within complex systems involving a range of organizations, the potential for further fragmentation of long-term and intricate care pathways is clear. However, there are some possible gains to be had; for example, more explicit funding mechanisms will help identify precious resources that are being misdirected and a greater focus on outcomes should help clinicians prioritize their efforts to improve their services. Overall, whether clinicians view this as a good or bad thing will depend on many factors; however, the fact is, it is happening and we need to ensure, to the best of our ability, that it works to the benefit of those who use our services. This means we will need to understand (and involve ourselves in) the commissioning process as much as possible, provide leadership in measuring quality and outcomes, and be active in our pursuit of better information and data quality.

In 2008, Health Minister Lord Darzi published the report of his review of the NHS. After 10 years of reform designed to increase capacity, the purpose of his review was to shift the focus more onto quality and personalization. Called 'High Quality Care for All' (Department of Health, 2008) it was developed through a process involving groups in each strategic health authority (SHA) area in England (which were clinically led) covering key elements of health care, including mental health. (SHAs were created by the government in 2002 to manage the local NHS on behalf of the secretary of state. There were originally 28 of them but in 2006 the number reduced to 10. They have managed the NHS locally and have been a key link between the Department of Health and the NHS.)

It highlighted variations in the quality of care and some of the future challenges to service provision including demographic changes, advances in treatment, rising expectations, and the changing nature of some diseases. It further emphasized the need for greater choice and personalization of services (including pilot personal health budgets), the need for quality standards, and greater accessibility of the best available evidence. In the latter two, it calls for the National Institute for Health and Clinical Excellence to take the lead role. It goes further, proposing systems for promoting innovation and also the measurement, publication, and funding of quality (which is described in terms of effectiveness, safety, and compassionate and personal care that recognizes the importance of preserving dignity). Although this report was wide-ranging, it emphasized the need for quality to be at the heart of health care provision and, among other things, highlighted professionalism. In particular, it suggested that there should be new programmes to develop leadership and that clinicians should have 'more control over budgets and HR decisions'. In other words, clinicians should develop the wherewithal to contribute more at a service management (as well as a clinical) level. To some, this will be welcomed with open arms; to others it might seem daunting. However, given the pace of change, the growth in the variety of services and interventions, the need to ensure mental health services thrive in an uncertain world and the need to retain a strong medical presence within them, there are key pointers as to how psychiatrists practising in England might best target much of their future effort.

With all the changes described so far, it is clear that the commissioning of services will assume greater importance and influence over what happens in future. For mental health services, there is evidence that this has so far been variable in its effects across the country (Glover, 2004) and there is a consequent need to ensure that key policy in this area is appropriately applied. At the time of writing, the current Government has signalled its intention to give General Practitioners the primary role in commissioning specialist health services. Clinicians have an important role to play in assessing local needs and shaping priorities. Their professional experience of delivering care, combined with their understanding of patients' needs, will be crucial to designing high-quality, personalised health and care services' (Department of Health, 2007). The extent to which psychiatrists will be able (and willing) to engage in commissioning processes will undoubtedly vary depending on local circumstances, but the profession as a whole should be prepared to offer expert advice and opinion whenever appropriate opportunities are apparent.

However, effective commissioning and service improvement will be dependent on good information and clear understanding of the effects of investment decisions. For mental health services in England, this currently presents a problem. Historically there has not been the level of investment in the architecture of information technology found in other fields of health care and there has arguably been a corresponding lack of accurate and detailed information available to service managers, planners, commissioners, and, of course, clinicians. For most teams of mental health professionals, information systems have been experienced as something of a black hole, sucking in whatever data staff provide, and giving little of value back. So for many, there have been few perceived advantages in taking an active interest in providing accurate and timely information.

This extends to the routine measurement of clinical outcomes. Although outcome measurement in mental health is not as straightforward as in some other specialist areas, it is certainly possible, there is a growing range of increasingly sophisticated measures (London School of Medicine and the Department of Health, 2009) and future investment is very likely to be increasingly dependent on the clear demonstration of clinical and quality improvement as well as improvements in patient experience and satisfaction. However, for this to work, there will be a need for clinical leadership; leadership to ensure that information systems fulfil their primary purpose in supporting clinical care first and also leadership to ensure that the practice of outcome measurement becomes core business for frontline teams. This does not necessarily have to come from psychiatrists but their background and training as doctors should make them well placed to do it. Furthermore, their interest in service improvement should mean that they understand the need for these foundations and how they should best be built.

Of course, the measurement of outcomes, whether by clinicians or self-reporting, provides only one dimension of quality and other indicators will help form a more complete picture. Indeed, in England we have a number of indicators sets with different provenance and purpose, which have been derived by different organizations; at a national level we will need to seek to achieve as much coherence and consistency across them as possible. Although the direction of travel is away from national targets, national and local indicators will continue to evolve and may be used in local target-setting in some areas. It is therefore important that clinicians are involved, along with others, in ensuring these evolve in a way that reflects continuous improvements in quality and minimizes any perverse incentives in the system.

Most psychiatrists in England are now very familiar with accelerating change in health and social care and the pace one can feel is deeply unsettling. Their professional training should have prepared them well to provide high-quality clinical assessment, judgement, treatment, and care but adapting to a changing landscape is difficult. Being adaptable and finding the space and time to think strategically about service development while struggling with the competing demands of a busy clinical schedule can be draining physically, intellectually, and emotionally. It is not surprising that resistance to further change is an issue for many who deliver treatment and care. What is disappointing is that the reasons underlying such conservatism sometimes remain unexplored by those who have key responsibility for planning and delivering new or realigned services.

As a profession, we have a responsibility to ensure that we do have the capacity and capability to engage with and (as appropriate) have a leading role in change. This has implications for the way we are trained and the way we practice. If we are to have time to be involved in quality improvement, service development and design, commissioning decisions, the clinical governance of care pathways, and 'more control over budgets and HR decisions' (see above), then something will probably have to give. Given the diversity in style of practice found within the profession (Kennedy & Griffiths, 2001) there does seem room for manoeuvre. If direct clinical work by psychiatrists can be more focused on circumstances where their particular knowledge and skills are essential, then more opportunities for strategic roles should emerge.

An example of how this could work is assessment. We are trained to undertake a detailed yet broad medical and psychosocial assessment from which to derive a formulation, diagnosis, and care plan. No other profession in the multidisciplinary team formally incorporates all those elements together in their assessments. So the question arises, should all people who come into contact with specialist mental health services see a psychiatrist first? For some services (e.g., many tertiary services) that may be entirely appropriate. However, the vast majority of people presenting with a mental health problems have all their treatment and help within primary care (Goldberg & Huxley, 1992). For most general mental health teams, the boundary between primary and secondary care is often vague and fluid, with the criteria for referral depending on a wide range of variables, not least of which is the extent of service and expertise available in GPs' practices. So at what point and for whom does an assessment by a psychiatrist become necessary? The point is that in this country, it is possible for psychiatrists to spend a large proportion of their time assessing a potentially overwhelming number of people referred from primary care (and, indeed, from other sources) if it is deemed essential for all to have such an assessment. However, the criteria would be arbitrary and constantly changing and whether it is the best use of their time is doubtful.

A better option would surely be to have psychiatrists play a lead role in the clinical governance of the assessment process by helping set agreed standards, ensuring others have the right training and proficiency, and by ensuring that there are appropriate arrangements for supervision and audit. In so doing, it should still be possible to select and see those for whom a psychiatric assessment is necessary and at the same time play a lead role in the development of the service. A significant number of consultant psychiatrists already function in such ways, and many have done so for a considerable number of years. Doubts have been expressed by others about the legitimacy of such styles of practice but the General Medical Council helpfully provided some clarification about the duties of doctors in multidisciplinary teams (General Medical Council, 2005), which should answer most concerns.

There may well be lessons here for psychiatrists who practise in other countries but much will depend on funding models for services and local capacity. For example, it may be difficult to achieve the necessary flexibility if other professions are scarce or poorly developed or if payment is primarily dependent on the number of patients seen by an individual.

Conclusion

All of this presents some significant challenges for the psychiatric profession. In addition to delivering our interventions and working to maximize the contribution of others, we will need to have our minds constantly looking to the future, aiming to shape, and adapt to change. We will need to take an active interest in the business side of health care as well as in clinical matters, but at the same time ensure we take an active role in the maintenance and improvement of quality and safety. Our practice will no doubt continue to evolve, and we will need constant renewal of our knowledge and skills to keep abreast of technical and organizational developments. Challenging though this may be, we have no choice if we are to play our full part in ensuring our population is as mentally healthy as possible. To do otherwise would arguably be to break our contract with society. If we succeed, we can transform public perceptions and expectations of mental health, provide the best services in the world and ensure that the voices of those who question the value of psychiatry grow ever fainter.

References

Bart's and the London School of Medicine and the Department of Health. (2009). *Outcomes Compendium: Helping You Select the Right Tools for Best Mental Health Care Practice in Your Field*. National Institute of Mental Health in England.

Department of Health. (1999). *National Framework for Mental Health: Modern Standards and Service Models*. London: Author.

Department of Health. (2000). *The NHS Plan: A Plan for Investment, a Plan for Reform*. London: Author.

Department of Health. (2007). *World Class Commissioning: Vision*. London: Author.

Department of Health. (2008). *High Quality Care for All: NHS Next Stage Review Final Report*. London: Author.

Department of Health. (2009a). *2008/2009 National Survey of Investment in Adult Mental Health Services*. London: Author.

Department of Health. (2009b). *New Horizons: Towards a Shared Vision for Mental Health – Consultation*. London: Author.

Department of Health. (2009c). *World Class Commissioning – An Introduction*. London: Department of Health.

Foresight Mental Capital and Wellbeing Project. (2008). *Final Project Report*.

General Medical Council. (October 2005). *Accountability in Multi-Disciplinary and Multi-Agency Mental Health Teams*.

Gijswijt-Hofstra, M., & Porter, R. (Eds). (1998). *Cultures of Psychiatry and Mental Health Care in Post-War Britain and Netherlands*. Clio Medica: Amsterdam.

Glover G. R. (2004). *Mental Health Funding in England*. Centre for Public Mental Health, Durham University.

Goldberg, D., & Huxley, P. (1992) *Common Mental Disorders: A Biosocial Model*. London: Routledge.

Kennedy, P., & Griffiths, H. W. (2001). General Psychiatrists Discovering New Roles for a New Era ... and Removing Work Stress *The British Journal of Psychiatry*, **179**, 283–285.

Laing, R. D. (1960). *The Divided Self: An Existential Study in Sanity and Madness*. Penguin Books.

Mental Health Act 1983, amended 2007.

Szasz, T. (1972). *The Myth of Mental Illness*. London: Paladin.

Szasz, T. (1976). *Schizophrenia: The Sacred Symbol of Psychiatry*. New York: Syracuse University Press

Chapter 14

Psychiatry's contract with society: revalidation and professionalism

Laurence Mynors-Wallis

Introduction

Revalidation is the process by which doctors in the United Kingdom will demonstrate to the General Medical Council (GMC) on a regular basis that they remain up to date and fit to practice. Revalidation will have three elements:

1 To confirm that licensed doctors practise in accordance with the GMC's generic standards as set out in *Good Medical Practice* (General Medical Council, 2006).

2 To confirm that doctors on the GMC Specialist Register or GP Register continue to meet the standards appropriate for their specialty. The Royal College of Psychiatrists has set out the standards for Psychiatry in *Good Psychiatric Practice*, third edition (2009).

3 To identify for further investigation and remediation poor practice where concerns remain despite local attempts at remediation.

The GMC has been planning to introduce revalidation for approximately 10 years. Although surveys regularly indicate that the public's trust and confidence in the medical profession is high, a series of high-profile scandals involving doctors led to concerns that the revalidation processes being contemplated were insufficiently robust. The criticism was voiced most eloquently by Dame Janet Smith in her Fifth Report following the Shipman Inquiry (Smith, 2004). She did not believe that the appraisal processes then proposed offered sufficient assurance for the public to have confidence in professional regulation. The current plans seek to ensure that both the public and the profession have confidence in revalidation, and it is neither seen as a bureaucratic stick with which to beat the profession nor a cosy consensus between colleagues from which the public are excluded.

The principles of revalidation were set out in the Chief Medical Officer for England's consultation documents *Good Doctors Safer Patients* adopted in the United Kingdom Government's White paper on professional regulation: *Trust Assurance and Safety – The Regulation of Health Professionals in the 21st Century* (HMSO, 2007b). These principles were summarized in *Medical Revalidation Principles and Next Steps* issued by the Department of Health for England (HMSO, 2009) – Revalidation:

- Must support doctors in meeting their personal and professional commitments to continually sustaining and developing their skills;
- should include within it a strong element of patient and carer participation and evaluation;
- should be seen primarily as supportive, focused on raising standards, not a disciplinary mechanism to deal with the small proportion of doctors who may cause concern;
- must include remediation and rehabilitation as essential elements of the process for the very few who struggle to revalidate, giving them help wherever possible;
- should be a continuing process, not an event every five years, so that problems can be identified and resolved quickly and effectively;
- should avoid bureaucracy, add value, and provide a reasonable level of reassurance to colleagues, employers, patients, and the public;
- should be introduced incrementally through piloting to ensure that it works well;
- should provide reasonably consistent assurance of standards across the United Kingdom, whatever the practice model;
- should be based on evidence drawn from local practice, with robust systems of clinical governance to support it; and
- will depend on the quality, consistency, and nature of appraisal to ensure the confidence of patients and doctors.

The Royal College of Psychiatrists in seeking to tailor revalidation for psychiatrists has built on the GMC and Department of Health principles and set out the following aims for revalidation:

- Revalidation must command the confidence of patients, the public, and the profession.
- Revalidation should facilitate improved practice for all members and fellows.

- The process should identify those whose practice falls below acceptable standards and give advice and monitoring to allow recertification to be reconsidered. There should be early warning of potential failure so remedial action can be taken.
- The process should allow those who are working to college standards to revalidate without undue difficulty or stress.
- There must be equity across the specialty – independent of differing areas of practice, working environments, and geographical location.
- Revalidation should be affordable and flexible, starting simple to allow further development.
- The process should incorporate as far as possible information already being collected in clinical work and use existing tools and standards where available.

The link between revalidation and professionalism

There can be few who doubt that the revalidation process will have a significant impact on being a doctor in the United Kingdom. Whatever parts of the process are emphasized, at the core of revalidation is the requirement for doctors to demonstrate that they continue to be fit to practise in an open, transparent, and accountable way. Continuing fitness to practise will no longer be left to the individual doctor's judgement or to informal, concerned discussions between colleagues and approaches to three wise men.

In considering the potential impact of revalidation on professionalism it is helpful to consider the practice of medicine over recent generations as a journey along a path from medicine as a vocation through medicine as a profession with the danger that the journey could end with medicine becoming a trade.

The generation of doctors for whom medicine was a vocation (and for many it may still be) worked very long hours, put the personal care of the patients above all other priorities, and in return received high levels of respect and trust. Most experienced little outside scrutiny of their practice. Many had little formal, continuing professional development after qualification, with ongoing learning in an apprenticeship model. I will not dwell on medicine as a profession as this is the focus of other chapters in the book. In brief, in moving from medicine as a vocation towards medicine as a profession, doctors while placing the care of patients as a priority recognize that other factors including family life are also important and that patient care may need to be shared with colleagues to allow decent working hours. There is an expectation that the working environment be satisfactory and that continuing professional development and additional qualifications are a key part of progressing within the profession. Medicine as a trade moves further towards a clarity about terms and conditions under which doctors work with clear hours for starting and finishing, rest breaks, working closely to protocols agreed by others, and working within clearly defined parameters. The competency-based training movement supports such a development with the requirement that medical practitioners meet specific competencies in their work with less emphasis on the holistic practice of being a doctor.

The regulation of medicine as a vocation was very much internal self-regulation with doctors setting themselves high standards often quite influenced by mentors and doctors they trained underneath. Many doctors continue to be hardworking, self-motivated, and self-critical. With medicine as a profession, the regulation moved toward Royal Colleges (colleagues) playing a key role with standards quantified and made explicit. Medicine as a trade could see employers setting standards and regulating the practice of the doctors they employ.

Revalidation should, if implemented appropriately, support the professionalism of doctors by ensuring that the key aspects of being a professional are valued and supported. There will be more explicit standard setting and more explicit monitoring of these standards. However, as the standards are set by the profession, professionalism should not be endangered. Revalidation, if implemented inappropriately, could hasten the journey of the profession on the path of vocation to trade by setting up bureaucratic hurdles and which devalue the overall practice of the doctor in favour of meeting revalidation targets.

How revalidation should support professionalism

At the time of writing this chapter, the details of what revalidation will mean for individual doctors are still being worked out between the General Medical Council, the Academy of Medical Royal Colleges, and the Department of Health. It is likely, however, that the revalidation process for all doctors will have broadly a similar structure in which they will be required to demonstrate information at appraisal in the areas of clinical practice, continuing professional development, feedback from patients and colleagues, and an appropriate response to complaints and serious untoward incidents.

Appraisal

All doctors will be required to collect a portfolio of evidence that will be reviewed at an annual appraisal. The standards for relicensing are those set out in good medical practice and the standards for recertification for psychiatrists are those set out in *Good Psychiatric Practice (3rd ed.)*. Revalidation is planned to take place on a five-yearly cycle and hence the necessary evidence to provide assurance about keeping up to date and fit to practise can be gathered over a five-year period.

The key process through which revalidation standards will be evidenced is appraisal. The NHS is piloting an enhanced appraisal process that will have both a summative and a formative component. The summative component of appraisal will involve looking back at what has been achieved and the formative part will be the agreeing of a personal development plan as to the way forward.

The appraisal process may continue to work in a similar way for those who are used to current NHS appraisal systems with practice being considered under the following headings.

  i. Good medical care
 ii. Maintaining good medical practice
iii. Working relationships with colleagues
 iv. Relations with patients
  v. Teaching and training
 vi. Probity
vii. Health

There will be an expectation that appraisers will have been trained to ensure that appraisal is delivered in a professional, fair, and transparent manner. The Royal College of Psychiatrists intends to establish an appraisal training system to ensure that there is an opportunity for psychiatrists to train using the recommended appraisal system linked to the specialist standards for psychiatry.

Doctors working in the UK National Health Service have been undertaking appraisal for many years. The focus of appraisal has been largely formative, that is, assisting the doctor in developing plans for the subsequent year to improve their practice. Although this will continue to be a focus of appraisal, revalidation will require a summative component to the appraisal process: looking back at what has been achieved and how successfully it has been achieved as well as looking forward. Although this might seem threatening and challenging to some, best practice in appraisal has always included a summative component. Indeed how can a doctor meaningfully plan to improve his or her practice without a clear understanding of what that practice has been? The distinction, therefore, between summative and formative components of appraisal is probably unhelpful. Appraisal needs to be considered as an opportunity for a doctor to reflect, with an experienced colleague, on their practice as a whole leading to a plan that will both develop and support the doctor in their work.

Demonstrating high-quality clinical practice

How doctors will demonstrate high-quality clinical practice will vary according to the branch of medicine the doctor is practising in. There are three broad categories in which most practice will be judged:

1. Workplace-based assessments
2. Clinical audit
3. Outcome measures

Workplace-based assessments

The Royal College of Psychiatrists is likely to recommend that the case-based discussion technique is used as a key component of appraisal. The system being proposed for those on the specialist register has been adapted from that used by trainees to meet the different requirements of more experienced doctors.

Case-based discussion provides the opportunity for a specialist psychiatrist to discuss the care of a real patient with a colleague. It provides an opportunity for the colleague to make an assessment of key clinical care standards set out in *Good Psychiatric Practice*. Case-based discussion evaluates what the doctor has actually done in practice. It has the advantage over a simple review of case notes in that the doctor being appraised has the opportunity to explain and clarify the information that is contained in the clinical records and provide appropriate clinical background.

The expectation is that at each case-based discussion, a judgement will be made as to whether the psychiatrist has satisfactorily met the standards being evaluated from *Good Psychiatric Practice*. Good points in the clinical care will be highlighted together with the identification of areas of improvement. Each area for improvement will then link to a personal development plan that will be followed up at appraisal.

It will be the responsibility of each consultant to ensure that an appropriate sample of the patients whom they are looking after is included in case-based discussion. To achieve this, it is likely that approximately two-thirds of case-based discussions should be chosen at random and the other third should be chosen by the psychiatrist being appraised.

Case-based discussion is not the only workplace assessment that might be of value in revalidation. If specialists wish to use other techniques, for example, direct observation of practice by a colleague, this information could be included in the evidence supporting satisfactory clinical care.

The danger with case-based discussion is that doctors may feel that their judgement is being critically scrutinized, which could potentially be illicit for a defensive response. In pilot work (involving 86 specialist psychiatrists) undertaken by the Royal College of Psychiatrists, funded by the Department of Health, the use of case-based discussion in revalidation was widely welcomed. The process can validate a doctor's practice as well as provide an opportunity for learning based on actual cases and actual decisions. These opportunities for many doctors ceased once they stopped training. Case-based discussion if done well should, for most doctors, provide an opportunity for demonstrating that they are meeting the best practice standards and in addition provide the opportunity for learning. Although case-based discussion involves talking about practice with a colleague, it is not a threat to professionalism; it is rather an opportunity to enhance professionalism.

Audit

Audit involves assessing the care of a number of patients in a specific area of practice rather than the care of a single patient as in case-based discussion. It is an impersonal process in which care is measured against a series of predetermined standards by reviewing case notes. Audit involves reviewing the care of a group of patients, it rarely involves examining the care provided by one doctor but rather a whole clinical team and reflects not only the individual care provided by a doctor but also the care provided by a team of clinicians within resources available. It is self-evident that it is easier to provide high-quality clinical care in well-staffed, well-resourced units. Notwithstanding these concerns, audit if done properly provides an opportunity for a doctor to demonstrate that he or she is a part of a team providing a satisfactory standard of care and clearly demonstrates where such care might be improved. Whether identified improvements are then the responsibility of the individual doctor or the responsibility of the organization or others will depend on the individual results.

Although some members of the profession have embraced audit as a tool for raising clinical standards and audit has led to significant improvements in care, particularly national audits such as the maternal deaths, and the suicide and homicide audit, many audits have been of poor quality and have not led to demonstrable patient benefit. The number and frequency of audits required for revalidation has yet to be determined. It is important, however, that the audits undertaken are clinically led, are of high quality, reflect significant areas of the clinician's practice, and robust action plans are put in place to remedy defects identified. Wherever possible, patients and carers should be involved both in the development of audit standards and reviewing the results. Audit provides an opportunity for members of the profession to work with patients in a collaborative way to improve outcomes.

The Royal College of Psychiatrists is drawing up a list of best practice audits that psychiatrists can use. This will avoid each individual psychiatrist reinventing the wheel and also allow the opportunity for benchmarking of results. Most clinicians will recognize that audits done well will lead to an improvement in care provided to patients and that the results may be used to enhance rather than criticize professional practice.

Outcome measures

As with audit, the enthusiasm with which the use of outcome measures has been embraced varies across the profession. Cardiovascular surgery has led the way in this regard with individual surgeon's mortality rates published and made available to patients. The Department of Health in England is implementing patient-reported outcome measures for certain designated areas of surgery, for example, hip and knee replacements, hernias, and varicose vein surgery. It is hoped that the national publication of these outcome measures will enhance good practice and provide patients with information to inform their decision making.

The Royal College of Psychiatrists is not recommending that outcome measures are to be used for revalidation at this stage. This reflects the fact that there are no nationally supported measures that allow for the fact that many psychiatric patients have long-term problems rather than a specific issue that will benefit from a specific intervention. It is the College's view, however, that psychiatrists should be considering, with colleagues, the use of appropriate outcome measures as a way of working with patients to determine the benefit or otherwise of interventions chosen. The National Institute for Mental Health in England (HMSO, 2008) has produced an outcomes compendium to assist in the choice of relevant measures. Using structured outcome measures to evaluate outcomes relevant to patients will be seen as an example of good practice for revalidation.

The open and transparent use of outcome measures should support professional practice. There are of course dangers in the process, in particular the potential for using outcome measures as a proxy for clinical performance. It may well be that even the best clinicians fail to get good outcomes for patients with complex and intractable problems.

Continuing professional development

The opportunity to participate in continuing professional development is a key plank of revalidation. All professionals will be expected to keep up with developments in their field of expertise. The Academy of Medical Royal Colleges has set out principles for continuing professional development:

1. An individual's continuing professional development (CPD) activities should be planned in advance through a personal development plan and should reflect and be relevant to his or her current and future profile of professional practice and performance. These activities should include CPD outside narrower specialty interests.
2. CPD should include activities both within and outside the employing institution, where there is one, and a balance of learning methods that include a component of active learning. Participants will need to collect evidence to record this process, normally using a structured portfolio cataloguing the different activities. This portfolio will be reviewed as part of appraisal and revalidation.
3. College/faculty CPD schemes should be available to all members and fellows and, at reasonable cost, to non-members and fellows who practise in a relevant specialty.
4. Normally, credits given by colleges/faculties for CPD should be based on one credit equating to one hour of educational activity. The minimum required should be an average of 50 per year. Credits for un-timed activities such as writing, reading, and e-learning should be justified by the participant or should be agreed between the provider(s) and college/faculty directors of CPD.
5. (i) Self-accreditation of relevant activities and documented reflective learning should be allowed and encouraged.
   (ii) Formal approval/accreditation of the quality of educational activities for CPD by colleges/faculties should be achieved with minimum bureaucracy and with complete reciprocity between colleges/faculties for all approved activities. The approval/accreditation process and criteria should be such as to ensure the quality and likely effectiveness of the activity.
6. Self-accreditation of educational activities will require evidence. This may be produced as a documented reflection. Formal CPD certificates of attendance at meetings will not be a requirement, but evidence of attendance should be provided, as determined by each individual college or faculty.
7. Participation in college-/faculty-based CPD schemes should normally be confirmed by a regular statement issued to participants that should be based on annually submitted returns and should be signed off at appraisal.
8. To quality assure their CPD system, colleges/faculties should fully audit participants' activities on a random basis. Such peer-based audit should

verify that claimed activities have been undertaken and are appropriate. Participants will need to collect evidence to enable this process.

9 Until alternative quality assurance processes are established, the proportion of participants involved in random audit each year should be of a size to give confidence that it is representative and effective. This proportion will vary according to the number of participants in a given scheme.

10 Failure to produce sufficient evidence to support claimed credits will result in an individual's annual statement being endorsed accordingly for the year involved and the individual being subsequently subject to audit annually for a defined period. Suspected falsification of evidence for claimed CPD activities will call into question the individual's fitness for revalidation and may result in referral to the GMC/GDC.

It will be a requirement of revalidation that doctors will demonstrate that they have met the standards for CPD as set by each of their colleges based on these 10 principles. The Royal College of Psychiatrists has adopted these principles in its most recent guidance to psychiatrists about continuing professional development. For those doctors in managed care organizations who find it difficult to identify time for CPD, the revalidation requirement for continuing professional development should support them in discussions with managers to identify suitable resources in terms of both time and money. For those doctors in non-managed care organizations, the requirements set clear expectations for them as to the proportion of their time spent in continuing professional development. Without doubt the public expect their psychiatrists to be up to date with developments in their field of practice.

Multi-source feedback from patients and colleagues

It is a GMC requirement that feedback is obtained for all doctors from colleagues and patients whether it be for relicensing or recertification. The expectation is that each doctor will use a GMC-approved multi-source feedback tool. It will be a recommendation that formal colleague and patient feedback occurs at least once every five years. The feedback should then be discussed with a colleague and an appropriate personal development plan drawn up to address any issues that arise.

The requirement for formal patient and colleague feedback is a minimum of one per five years and assumes that no significant concerns have arisen. If significant concerns have been picked up by multi-source feedback, a second multi-source feedback should be undertaken in the five-year cycle, following appropriate action by the doctor concerned.

Multi-source feedback from colleagues and patient feedback allow psychiatrists to meet several of the standards for good medical and good psychiatric practice concerned with teamwork, working with colleagues, and communicating with patients. The Royal College of Psychiatrists has devised a feedback tool: ACP360 specifically for psychiatrists (Lelliott et al., 2008). Using this tool will enable psychiatrists to be compared with their UK colleagues and provide a useful benchmark against which to draw up appropriate actions.

Obtaining structured feedback from both colleagues and patients is a useful technique to guard against arrogance and poor practice. In many cases the results will validate a doctor's performance. For some doctors, however, the feedback will identify concerns about practice they were not aware of. Although this form of scrutiny might be initially painful, the good (and professional) doctor will welcome such feedback to improve practice. As with many other areas of revalidation, feedback should be provided by a colleague in a structured and supportive setting with the focus on improving practice rather than criticism.

Complaints and serious untoward incidents

It is expected that psychiatrists will reflect upon complaints and on serious untoward incidents involving patients in their care and identify not only good practice but also areas for improvement. The areas for improvement will form part of a personal development plan and be signed off through the appraisal process.

Managed care organizations may provide detailed information from incident reporting systems: for example, violent episodes, falls, deliberate self-harm that may be used to provide evidence of cooperating with such systems (which is good practice), and also work undertaken by the individual doctor to deal with any issues raised by such reporting systems.

A structured approach to management of complaints and serious untoward incidents will protect the psychiatrist against criticism and also demonstrate that the doctor has a reflective, open approach to complaints and serious untoward incidents. A good (and professional) doctor should use such incidents as an opportunity for learning and development.

Non-clinical practice

Many psychiatrists spend a significant proportion of their time in non-clinical practice including academic work, both teaching and research, management activities, and medico-legal work. The Academy of Medical Royal Colleges is drawing up guidelines as to how such non-clinical work could be appropriately assessed at appraisal. Examples of relevant evidence could be as follows:

- *Teaching.* Evidence to show that psychiatrists involved in teaching are meeting the standards of good psychiatric practice would include information about the content of a teaching course together with feedback from students.
- *Research.* Evidence of compliance with good medical and psychiatric practice would include information about meeting national and local research governance arrangements.
- *Management.* Details of management activities and projects involving patient benefit in which the individual doctor has played a significant part could be included.

How concerns will be dealt with

The expectation is that the majority of doctors will demonstrate satisfactory practice at appraisal. Each appraisal will result in a personal development plan that will be reviewed in subsequent years with the aim of improving practice. For most doctors no significant concerns will be identified. There will be a small group of doctors, for whom either through appraisal or through other mechanisms, concerns are identified. For most of these doctors, the concerns will be managed through a clear plan aimed at remedying the identified problems. This will be reviewed either at appraisal or by another identified mechanism. The expectation for most of these doctors is that within the five-year cycle of revalidation, concerns will have been appropriately dealt with.

At the end of a five-year process, each doctor will have had five appraisals. Satisfactory completion of five appraisals and the appropriate resolution of any identified concerns should lead to a responsible officer (HMSO, 2007a) making a recommendation to the GMC that the doctor be revalidated for a further five years. The details of this process remain, at the time of writing this chapter, uncertain. The roles and responsibility of the responsible officer have been subject to a consultation at the department of health and a further consultation document is expected.

In considering the link between revalidation and professionalism, it is important that this final stage of the process occurs in the same spirit as appraisal and the components of appraisal, that is, with transparent standards, strong involvement from colleagues within a supportive framework. It has been suggested that employers may be responsible for the final sign-off of revalidation. The concern about this suggestion is that employers may bring other factors into their decision making, for example, whether the doctor is seen as 'difficult' rather than there being a clear focus on the standards set in good medical practice and good psychiatric practice.

Conclusion

The proposals for revalidation in the United Kingdom may be seen by doctors either as a threat or as a support to professionalism. The threat comes from the potential of involving doctors in bureaucratic tick box exercises that seem to have little relevance to their practice. This will not only put off individuals coming into the profession but will also demoralize hard-working clinicians. A more optimistic view is that the processes of revalidation will support professionalism by identifying what it means to be a good doctor, allowing doctors to evidence good practice at appraisal and ensuring that sufficient time and attention is given to allowing the doctor to evaluate and improve their professional practice. The Royal College of Psychiatrists is working hard with the other Medical Royal Colleges to ensure that revalidation sits firmly within the principles described at the beginning of the chapter and that the aims that the Royal College of Psychiatrists has set for revalidation are met.

References

General Medical Council. (2006). *Good Medical Practice*. London: General Medical Council.

HMSO. (2007a). *Health and Social Care Bill*. London: HMSO.

HMSO. (2007b). *Trust Assurance and Safety. The Regulation of Health Professionals in the 21st Century*. London: HMSO.

HMSO. (2008). *Mental Health Outcomes Compendium*. London: National Institute of Mental Health in England, London: HMSO.

HMSO. (2009). *Medical Revalidation Principles and Next Steps*. London: HMSO.

Lelliott, P., Williams, R., Mears, A., et al. (2008) Questionnaires for 360-degree assessment of consultant psychiatrists. *British Journal of Psychiatry*, **193**, 156–160.

Royal College of Psychiatrists. (2009). *Good Psychiatric Practice* (3rd ed). Royal College of Psychiatrists.

Smith, D. J. (2004).*The Shipman Inquiry: Fifth Report; Safeguarding Patients, Lessons from the Past and Proposals for the Future*. London: HMSO.

Chapter 15

Professionalism and medicine: a managerial perspective

Naaz Coker

At the heart of all definitions of medical professionalism is the ethos of patient service and integrity of values, actions, and behaviours. Simultaneously this is coupled with concepts of leadership, self-regulation, autonomy, and privilege. It was interesting to note that the 2005 Royal College of Physicians report, *Doctors in Society: Medical Professionalism in a Changing World,* talked about 'serious' failures in medical leadership. It stated, 'While there are many leaders within medicine, there is little leadership of medicine as a whole.' Where is this leadership going to come from? Will we recognize it if we see it? Can it be learnt?

As a manager, I recognize that good medicine is not just about knowledge and expertise. Doctors have to practise in an environment of uncertainty; solutions are not always apparent and wisdom and judgement become part and parcel of medical decision-making. It therefore becomes extremely important that decisions are made and conveyed to patients in a way that both they and their families understand the philosophy and the treatment underpinning the medical care proposed. Although the public still hold doctors in high regard, they also know what poor professionalism does to them. Medical professionalism therefore must combine up-to-date professional knowledge and skills as well as respect, compassion, integrity, and collaboration.

These challenges are shared by health systems globally. In the UK National Health Service (NHS), which is government controlled, there is often a tendency for the medical profession to blame politicians, government, or senior managers for all the changes and challenges facing them. Yet the social, technological, and financial changes are affecting health professionals worldwide and certainly all health systems in the western world are affected by these changes. Professionalism in all health systems will need to be redefined in light of global changes in economy, public expectations, and new models of health care delivery systems.

The General Medical Council's (GMC) most recent edition of *Good Medical Practice* (GMC, 2006), which 'sets out the principles and values on which good practice is founded describe these principles as medical professionalism in action'. These duties are certainly very patient-centred and emphasize the importance of working in partnership with patients (see Box 15.1).

Box 15.1 Duties of a doctor

Good Medical Practice sets out the duties of a doctor as follows:

> Patients must be able to trust doctors with their lives and health. To justify that trust you must show respect for human life and you must:

- Make the care of your patient your first concern
- Protect and promote the health of patients and the public
- Provide a good standard of practice and care
  - Keep your professional knowledge and skills up to date
  - Recognize and work within the limits of your competence
  - Work with colleagues in the ways that best serve patients' interests
- Treat patients as individuals and respect their dignity
  - Treat patients politely and considerately
  - Respect patients' right to confidentiality
- Work in partnership with patients
  - Listen to patients and respond to their concerns and preferences
  - Give patients the information they want or need in a way they can understand
  - Respect patients' right to reach decisions with you about their treatment and care
  - Support patients in caring for themselves to improve and maintain their health
- Be honest and open and act with integrity
  - Act without delay if you have good reason to believe that you or a colleague may be putting patients at risk
  - Never discriminate unfairly against patients or colleagues
  - Never abuse your patients' trust in you or the public's trust in the profession.

You are personally accountable for your professional practice and must always be prepared to justify your decisions and actions.

The NHS Constitution, long-awaited and finally published in January 2009 (Department of Health, 2009) is a significant document that highlights the purpose, principles, and values of the NHS and sets out a clear set of rights, responsibilities, and pledges for staff, patients, and the public who use and work in the NHS in England.

Professionalism is at the heart of the Constitution seeking a balance between individual roles and responsibilities and the responsibilities of the whole health care system in which staff operate. In its introductory paragraph, the Constitution states as follows (Department of Health, 2009):

> The NHS belongs to the people. It is there to improve our health and well-being, supporting us to keep mentally and physically well, to get better when we are ill and, when we cannot fully recover, to stay as well as we can to the end of our lives. It works at the limits of science – bringing the highest levels of human knowledge and skill to save lives and improve health.
>
> It touches our lives at times of basic human need, when care and compassion are what matter most.

Although all definitions of medical professionalism emphasize the need for doctors to strive for excellence, integrity, altruism, and compassion, the NHS Constitution takes the challenge a whole step further into a set of legal rights around access to services, quality of care in clean and safe environment, partnership in design, and choice of services and appropriate response to complaints. A big theme of the Constitution is driving the quality agenda forward. For example, it says that care should be provided in safe, clean environments and that it should be based on best practice. It pledges that the NHS will collect more information about quality and share best practice on quality of care and treatment. It also pledges that decisions about services and treatments will be made in a clear and transparent way.

Quality was also at the core of the recent Lord Darzi's report *High Quality Care for All* (Darzi, 2009). The report describes quality as 'patient experience, clinical effectiveness, and patient safety'. Clinical leadership and professionalism are featured strongly in the report with emphasis on clinicians and their teams being responsible for quality outcomes as well as managing budgets. Lord Darzi's reforms provide a long-term vision for the NHS and although there are many critics of his strategic direction, one cannot argue that his direction for the change in the culture of the medical profession is to be highly commended.

Psychiatric professionalism in this context places a significant challenge for both professionals and the NHS as a system. It can no longer rely on good will and integrity of individuals. Doctors will need to learn about a new professionalism in their medical training. Medical curriculum will need to incorporate the new scientific content as well as the behavioural and leadership skills that will be required to practice it in an environment where accountability and measurement of performance has become paramount. Hilton and Slotnick (2005) set out six domains in which professionalism is manifested: an ethical practice, reflection and self-awareness, responsibility for actions, respect for patients, teamwork, and social responsibility. To this I would add leadership, communication, and resource management.

It is inevitable that there will be obstacles in delivery and learning of professionalism. These are illustrated in Table 15.1.

Paternalism

Paternalism is associated with doctors telling their patients what is good for them, without always considering the needs and wishes of the patients and/or their families. The concept has traditionally been based on a 'father–child' relationship where the father (the doctor) armed with knowledge and expertise treated the child (the patient) as ignorant and unable to understand his or her illness or its treatment. Even 20 years ago, patients trusted their doctors completely as they had confidence in the knowledge and skills of their doctors and believed that medical decisions were made in their best interest. Although the paternalistic relationship had good intentions and the doctors always thought that they acted in the best interest of the patient, in today's world of 'expert patients', paternalism has acquired a negative connotation. The era of 'doctor knows best' is definitely at an end.

Today people know more about health matters, and there is easy access to clinical information from the Internet. There is also intense public interest generated by the media in health matters, and the expectation of patients is increasingly high. Patients want to be well informed and want an open relationship with their doctors. Many want to be involved in making decisions about their treatment.

Anecdotally, clinicians generally and especially doctors, are finding it hard to come to terms with what they feel is a questioning of their status, skills, and

Table 15.1 What gets in the way of professionalism?

---
1 Paternalism
2 Secrecy
3 Arrogance
4 Lack of respect for patients and public
5 Discrimination
6 Loss of moral compass
7 Conflict with management
8 Lack of leadership
---

professional autonomy. They have to learn to embrace partnership and collaboration as a normal way of working in the future.

Lack of transparency and accountability

There have been major concerns about the lack of transparency in clinical practice. A case in point was the public inquiry into the Bristol Royal Infirmary children's cardiac services in 1998 when two cardiac surgeons and the chief executive who was medically qualified were found guilty of professional misconduct by the GMC. The inquiry report (July 2001) is a mandatory read for all health professionals. It is described as:

> An account of people who cared greatly about human suffering, and were dedicated and well-motivated. Sadly, some lacked insight and their behaviour was flawed. Many failed to communicate with each other, and to work together effectively for the interests of their patients. There was a lack of leadership, and of teamwork.
>
> In another part of the report, it states: Bristol was awash with data. There was enough information from the late 1980s onwards to cause questions about mortality rates to be raised both in Bristol and elsewhere had the mindset to do so existed. Little, if any, of this information was available to the parents or to the public. Such information as was given to parents was often partial, confusing and unclear. For the future, there must be openness about clinical performance. Patients should be able to gain access to information about the relative performance of a hospital, or a particular service or consultant unit.

The inquiry exposed many deficiencies in both individuals and the organization, and lack of transparency and accountability were two of the key aspects highlighted in the report. It is shocking that this was not exposed by clinicians who were aware of the unusually high mortality rates and who opted to 'look the other way'. There are many such examples everyday in the health system and although clinical governance and reporting of performance outcomes is addressing it to some extent, there is still the 'closing of the ranks' that undermines the trust between the public and the professional.

Arrogance

Although majority of doctors cannot be described as arrogant, there are, nevertheless, still significantly large numbers of doctors who exhibit arrogant behaviours that undermine their professionalism. 'Throwing the toys out of the pram' is an expression that is often associated with the behaviour of some specialists in the NHS. Examples of such behaviour include hiding behind notions of 'clinical freedom' and autonomy when challenged by managers, to ignoring and/or sabotaging decisions made collectively by colleagues and managers.

Arrogance, however, is not just confined to the individual. System arrogance can also block professionalism. An organizational culture that does not facilitate professionals to deliver good quality care by lack of investment in training and development or good quality information systems can easily hamper a professional approach to patient care. A good example of this was provided by the investigation at Mid Staffordshire NHS Foundation Trust (Healthcare Commission, 2009) undertaken following concerns about apparently high mortality rates and poor standards of care. The investigation report stated:

> We found that, when challenged, neither the trust nor individual consultants could produce an accurate record of their clinical activity or outcomes for patients. This meant that we could not analyse the volume of surgical work and its outcomes.
>
> The nurses in A&E had not had enough training and development, and leadership had been weak. Patients often waited for medication, pain relief and wound dressings. There were delays in scanning patients out of normal hours. The most senior surgical doctor in the hospital after 9 pm was often junior and inexperienced. There were too few consultants to provide on call cover all day, every day. There were too few middle grade doctors. The junior doctors were not adequately supervised, and were often put under pressure to make decisions quickly in order to avoid breaches of the target for all patients to be seen and moved from A&E in four hours.

Lack of respect for patients and public

All surveys of patient experiences highlight respect and dignity as one of the cornerstones of good clinical care; indeed they are two of the key values of the NHS and yet the NHS fails in this area as a system and through its many staff patients frequently complain about the way they are spoken to by staff on the telephone or face to face, or the way their needs for information and explanation are dismissed. Many feel that they are perceived as a statistic rather than as equal human beings with rights. Patients want and expect to be treated with respect as partners in the decision-making process about their care. This may not always be possible in all cases, and the professional may have to make decision in the best interest of the patient. Nevertheless the imperative must be to uphold the standards of dignity and compassion at all times.

Discrimination

Discrimination results when an individual or a group is able to act on their prejudices in a way that discriminates (negatively or positively) against another individual or group. The result of negative discrimination can be a denial of rights to services, resources, or respect. These prejudices are commonly around differences in age, ethnicity, religion, social class, and gender.

Much has been written about discrimination in the health service and its impact on health outcomes of groups who are discriminated against (Coker, 2001; Smaje, 1995). Discrimination, in all its forms, dehumanizes people, and it is well known that this generates a sense of powerlessness in people, which is associated with increased prevalence of illnesses, both physical and mental. The record of the NHS in removing discrimination is mixed. There are regular reports in the press about NHS being racist, ageist, and so on. One cannot be complacent about this. Doctors should challenge discriminatory practices in all its forms. Challenging the attitudes, behaviours, and actions of staff and colleagues is essential if we are to wipe out discriminatory practices in the NHS.

Loss of moral compass

Practising ethical medicine underpins medical professionalism. A professional code of ethics provides the essential moral compass for the delivery of good quality patient care. Losing moral compass for an individual can include accepting financial gifts from pharmaceutical companies to condoning (or ignoring) incompetent practices of colleagues.

Losing moral compass was epitomized by Enron, the energy giant that was once the seventh largest company in the United States and its collapse in late 2001 was the largest corporate failure in US history. It was frequently named as one of America's 10 topmost admired corporations and best places to work, and its board was acclaimed one of the US' best five, according to *Fortune* magazine. And yet, Enron became the largest bankruptcy reorganization in American history, and was described as the biggest audit failure. In an interview after the collapse, its finance director said, 'We lost our moral compass.'

There are similar instances in the NHS too. Maidstone and Tunbridge Wells NHS Trust (Healthcare Commission, 2007) and Mid Staffordshire hospital NHS Trust (Maidstone, 2009) were criticized for their poor hygiene standards, and ultimately poor management that resulted in poor standards of care. It was claimed that closed cultures, which failed to admit and deal with things going wrong were to blame for their failures.

Conflict with management

Conflict between clinicians and managers is well known and often results from, misinformation, misunderstanding of roles, and miscommunication. Refusal to see the other's perspective causes feelings to run high, egos get threatened, and the situations become disruptive. Clinicians getting involved in the management of their organizations have gone some way to alleviate this but there is a long way to go. Clinicians have to appreciate the challenge of delivering care with scarce resources, the need for integrating efficiency with patient safety and good quality care. These are not mutually exclusive parameters. The changing health care environment with commissioners demanding high-quality care and measurable performance outcomes that are benchmarked against other providers require clinicians to work alongside the managers so they can collectively meet the needs of their patients and deliver safe, effective, and compassionate care.

Lack of leadership

Leadership in one of the most complex systems in the world, such as the NHS, will always remain a huge challenge. Leaders in a health system have to deal simultaneously with pressures of managing budgets, meeting deadlines, inspiring reluctant colleagues, ensuring safe systems of work, and aligning multiple interests and agendas. Notwithstanding many clinicians who have, in recent years, demonstrated excellent leadership, the medical profession generally has shown a lack of leadership in engaging with the wider dilemmas of NHS management. Leadership skills can be learnt if there is a sense of purpose and commitment. Managers need clinicians to work with them and not against them.

Lack of empathy

Many patients' complaints refer to lack of empathy on the part of their doctor; sometimes this is a result of poor communication skills and at other times it is about professional dominance where the patient is not treated as an equal human being. My own experience as a patient has been very mixed; when the doctor has shared a story or a joke while explaining about my treatment plan, it has gone a long way towards making me feel better than when I was treated as a 'damaged hip' that needed fixing with little empathy. At the heart of this is the nature of the patient–doctor interaction. It is surprising to me that in spite of communications skills being a core part of medical training today, there are still so many clinicians who do not pay sufficient attention to compassionate interaction.

Future needs and challenges

Understanding the changing environment

The health care environment is always changing and is about to change again as the economic environment gets tougher and a general election approaches. There is no getting away from the fact that the NHS is a politicized environment and will remain so, at least for the next few years as no UK political party is willing to either privatize or remove it from government control. The previous Labour government introduced many new initiatives, including separating commissioning and provision, creation of foundation trusts, introduction of private sector providers in the system, delivery of high quality care in a tough financial climate, the need for efficiency and value for money, and patient safety; these are all challenges health care professionals had to address. Many of these changes were designed to improve the patient experience and the quality of patient care. The new Coalition Government of Conservatives and Liberal Democrats will introduce further changes which, once again, the managers and the professional in the service will have to take on board.

Doctors cannot bury their heads in the sand and pretend that either the change is not happening or will go away. They have to acknowledge the reality of working in a complex system such as the NHS; there are no magic formulas or guidebooks to control or manage this system. They have to understand the context within which they practice, work together with their managerial and clinical colleagues to develop values and guiding principles, and co-create a system that will facilitate the best possible patient care in an environment that is clean, safe, and respectful of individual dignity.

Leadership and partnership with management

Defining good leadership will always be a challenge – it is the ultimate motherhood and apple pie theme. What does it take to bring together disparate groups of individuals, professionals, teams, and occupational groups and unite them to achieve a common goal? How do you balance the need of the individual against the need of the collective system? These are some of the ongoing leadership challenges and yet we do know and recognize good leadership when it is present in our working environments. In my experience good clinical leadership keeps an eye on the bigger picture while working at an individual level. The nature of the relationships, be it with patients or colleagues or with the organization is the essence of good leadership. Leadership is not about command and control over others but working with others to achieve the best solution. The focus on hierarchies and occupational or specialty divisions just get in the way of forming productive relationships necessary for the delivery of common goals. It is not the specialties that matter but how the people within the specialties work together to make the patient experience a positive one.

Effective clinical leadership requires development of a minimum set of knowledge and skills such as the following:

1 An understanding of the organizational and financial structures of the NHS
2 ability to contribute to a strategic vision that is in the best interest of the patients, public, and staff
3 working in partnership with patients

4 delivering the business plans
5 effective communication skills
6 understanding the nature of accountability and performance management
7 effective teamwork that requires respect and understanding of the roles of all professionals
8 ability to resolve inter- and intra-professional conflicts.

Leadership skills have to be taught and learnt. It is wrong to assume that a bright, articulate, and expert clinician will automatically be able to assume a leadership role without any training. At St George's Healthcare Trust, for example, a clinical leadership programme is currently in progress for all the clinical directors and the clinical leaders in the organization.

Equity and human rights

Human rights are 'basic rights to humane dignified treatment and things I should have access to simply because I am a human being' (*Mental Health Service User*; Department of Health, 2007)

The need to ensure justice and equity and respect for human rights are enshrined in the Human Rights Act 1998. A human rights-based approach to health care delivery was highlighted in a Department of Health publication in 2007 'Human Rights in health care – a framework for local action', which provided a framework for embedding human rights in the design and delivery of services.

The five key principles of the 'Human Rights Based Approach' (HRBA) outlined in the document are as follows:

- putting human rights at the heart of policy and planning,
- empowering staff and patients with knowledge skills and organizational leadership and commitment to achieve human rights-based approaches,
- enabling meaningful involvement and participation of all key stakeholders,
- ensuring accountability throughout the organization,
- non-discrimination and attention to vulnerable groups.

These could be the principles for new professionalism in medicine too. Many marginalized groups do not have access to health services and even when they do eventually get access, they are met with a barrage of discriminating behaviours and actions, sometimes unintentional and occasionally intentional. However, equity is not just about protecting the rights of marginalized groups but about protecting the rights of everyone.

Research has shown that the application of human rights principles, for example dignity and respect can help to improve a patient's experience and Quality of care and will inevitably lead to improved outcomes.

(Audit Commission, 2003)

It is widely assumed that delivering the equity agenda will consume more resources; however, there is no evidence to support this. In my experience equity of care results in better outcomes for all which in the long term, reduces the cost of healthcare provision.

Living the values

The NHS was founded on a common set of values, the key ones being comprehensive service free at the point of delivery and equal care for all. More recently the NHS Constitution has redefined those values as follows:

- Respect and dignity
- Commitment to quality of care
- Compassion
- Improving lives
- Working together for patients
- Everyone counts.

Some organizations, such as my own, St George's Healthcare NHS Trust, describes its values as shown in Box 15.2.

Whatever we say about values they will always remain as words and exhortations until all staff learn to 'live' those values and challenge each other when they are violated. These values should form the ethical codes underpinning the services doctors and all staff collectively provide. Ethical and moral

---

Box 15.2 Living the values

We will
- treat all people with respect and dignity
- deliver care in partnership with others
- continually strive for clinical excellence
- ensure probity and transparency in spending public money
- be an exemplary employer
- be committed to excellence in education, training and research
- be open and honest with each other and those outside the organization

questions about behaviours and relationship are not religious concepts but fundamental to how we engage with each other and the public.

Thinking whole system

Whole systems thinking is a concept or philosophy that is based on the belief that organizations and especially a complex one such as the NHS comprise a whole series of connected sub-systems that do not and cannot work in isolation. Any change or action in one part of the system will affect another part of the system. Therefore to understand the whole, we have to understand the relationship and connections in each part of the system.

The Sufi parable of the five blind men and the elephant provides a good illustration. When asked to describe the elephant, one, feeling the tail described the elephant as a rope; the second feeling the leg described it as a tree trunk; the third feeling the side of the body described it as a leather-covered wall; the fourth feeling the ear described it as a bird with huge wing and the fifth feeling the trunk described it as a serpent. Knowing only the parts and blind to the whole, they never understood the whole animal.

Applying this analogy to the National health service implies that one can similarly remain blind to the needs of the whole service and can be in danger of drawing very incomplete and inaccurate decisions based on knowledge or needs of one specialty or directorate in isolation. To understand the whole professionals we have to examine and understand all the linkages and interactions between the various individuals, professional groups, and other players who make up the health system. This is critical in a professional setting. The sad story of Baby P (Siddique et al., 2008) illustrates this most aptly. Baby P born in 2006 was found dead in 2007 aged 17 months with horrendous injuries, having suffered neglect and abuse at the hands of his mother and stepfather. During his short life, he had over 60 contacts with the health and social care system and yet all the individual professionals (GPs, social services staff, hospital staff, health visitors, and the police) involved did not connect their stories to get the whole picture. This, in my opinion was a significant failure of professionalism on the part of all the professionals involved and a classic case of whole system failure.

Conclusion

I suspect that some of the things I have said may be a repetition of what others may have said before me. However, I have drawn from my clinical and managerial experiences to convey my views about medical professionalism and hope that I have provided some new thinking in how doctors can engage with the health system and its organization. Doctors not only have to be multi-skilled and work in multidisciplinary teams; they increasingly have to understand the business of health. This does not take away their specific and specialist expertise. Developing expertise and excellence in their field is critical but it also has to be coupled with societal and political considerations. None of us works in a vacuum and recognizing the linkages and connectedness of the system becomes a professional prerogative.

The emphasis on excellence in clinical care, observance of ethical standards with respect to dignity, and compassion accompanied by a holistic model of health and well-being is what characterizes medical professionalism. It also places a clear responsibility on NHS organizations, as a system to help and facilitate clinicians to become professional. As a chair of a large teaching hospital, I accept the responsibility of ensuring that the trust and its systems should strive to make it easy for all staff to deliver care to the highest professional standards; but in return I expect the medical staff to be the ultimate role models for the new professionalism required in today's rapidly changing environment.

References

Audit Commission. (September 2003). *Human Rights: Improving Public Service Delivery*. Audit Commission.

Coker, N. (2001). *Racism in Medicine: An Agenda for Change*. King's Fund.

Darzi, A. (2008). *High Quality Care for All: NHS Next Stage Review Final Report*. London: Department of Health.

Department of Health. (2007). *Human Rights in Healthcare – A Framework for Local Action*. London: Department of Health, COI.

Department of Health. (2009). *NHS Constitution Produced by COI for the Department of Health*. London: Department of Health.

General Medical Council, (2006). *Good Medical Practice*. GMC website. Retrieved 2 July 2010 from www.gmcuk.org/guidance/good_medical_practice/.

Healthcare Commission. (2001). *The Inquiry into the management of care of children receiving complex hear surgery at the Bristol Royal Infirmary*. London: Healthcare Commission.

Hilton, S. R., & Slotnick, H. B. (2005). Proto-professionalism: How professionalisation occurs across the continuum of medical education. *Medical Education*, **39**, 58–65.

Maidstone, T. (2009). *Wells Report Healthcare Commission. Investigation into Mid Staffordshire NHS Foundation Trust*. London: Healthcare Commission.

Royal College of Physicians. (2005). *Doctors in Society: Medical Professionalism in a Changing World*. Report of a Working Party of the Royal College of Physicians of London. London: Author.

Siddique et al. (1 December 2008). Baby P case: Key officials: guardian.co.uk.

Smaje, C(1995). *Health Race and Ethnicity*. King's Fund Institute.

Chapter 16

Changing professionalism

Edwin Borman

Introduction

The medical profession is being challenged as never before. This reflects a historic shift in power that will have consequences as great as the political and industrial revolutions that brought power to the professional classes. Empowered consumers or – in the context of health care – patients increasingly will demand an input in decision-making at all levels of the health care system.

This may be considered as threatening by a profession that perceives itself as losing power through this social change. However, it is argued here that only by embracing this opportunity, more fully to align itself with the patients that it serves, will the medical profession be able to develop a new professionalism, appropriate for this new century.

Professionalism

Professions can be defined by a limited number of characteristics and, in many cases, it is possible to chart the development of a profession by the achievement, as milestones, of these.

The first to occur is the establishment of a specific *area of practice*, determined by the work done, or the service provided by practitioners. This may be through the formal recognition of an existing craft, as occurred with Medicine, or through the establishment of a wholly new practice, such as has occurred in the computing sector.

The next step is that of *organization*, a visual testament to which can be seen in the Place de Petit Sablon in Brussels, where each of the 48 statues that surround the garden commemorate a particular sixteenth century craft and its guild. In the context of health care in the United Kingdom, an analogous process occurred, and continues to occur, as is demonstrated by the Medical Royal Colleges, the first of which to receive its charter, in 1518, being the Royal College of Physicians of London. The characteristic of organization can also be seen in the establishment, in 1832, of the British Medical Association (BMA), the trade union and professional association for doctors.

The third characteristic of a profession is that of *education*, through which students are trained to become practitioners, and practitioners may continue their training, thereby developing more advanced areas of competence. In addition to maintaining appropriate standards in education, the establishment, in 1858, of the General Medical Council (GMC) was to deliver the fourth requirement, *registration*: the means of confirming, to members of the public, who is a qualified practitioner – and, hence, who is not.

The GMC also became responsible for the fifth characteristic, the *regulation* of practitioners: dealing with those doctors who do not practise in accordance with the required standards. This too has been an area that has seen evolution, with consideration of a complaint regarding a potential deficiency in a doctor's fitness to practice initially only being considered owing to their conduct, later their health, and, only as recently as 1995, their performance.

It is through the delivery, over many years – by individual practitioners, of defined standards of practice, and by the profession as a whole – of each the above five characteristics, that the sixth characteristic is achieved, that of a specific professional *ethos*.

Professionalism – challenged

It can be seen therefore that, through the continuing delivery of these characteristics the 'great medical institutions' – the Royal Colleges, the BMA, and the GMC – have played, and continue to play, a crucial role in the development and maintenance of Medicine, as a profession, in the United Kingdom.

Historically, this recognition of medicine as a valued profession has also shaped what can be described as an unwritten 'social contract' between the public, the state, and practitioners. To a large extent, this unwritten contract determines the status and reward accorded to doctors.

However, as evidenced by the often-quoted phrase of George Bernard Shaw, 'All professions are conspiracies against the laity' (*The Doctor's Dilemma*, 1911), for many years, this social contract has been subject to a continuing process of negotiation, both implicit and explicit. The last 20 years have been a particularly tumultuous period in this regard, during which the relationship between the medical profession and society has been subject to considerable review. In the case of the medical profession, there have been many specific reasons why this should have occurred: medical 'scandals'; the availability of resources for healthcare, and; changes in policies for the National Health Service. However, given that a similar process of renegotiation of the 'social contract' is also occurring for many other professions, it is clear that greater, historically significant powers are at play.

Power has shifted and is shifting again

The statues in the centre of the Place de Petit Sablon commemorate Count Egmont and his cousin, Count de Hoorns, noblemen who were executed during the religious power struggles that swept through Europe during the sixteenth century. Although religions and states warred, the professions survived, prospered, and prepared for even greater political change.

We all are familiar with the view of history that, starting in 1789, in France, the near-monopoly hold on power of royalty and clergy, through a series of political revolutions, was swept aside by 'the masses'. To those forces were added the considerable social and economic changes of the industrial revolution. However, this interpretation – that wilfully may have been encouraged – hides the fact that it was not the working classes that were the primary beneficiaries of these revolutions, but the professional classes. Consider who now governs Britain, Europe, the World, and it is clear that the history of the last 250 years has been the history of the rise of the professional classes.

However, were we to analyse the times within which we now are living, with a similar focus on who wields power, we might consider that the world is entering a new phase, in which ordinary citizens are becoming a more significant, perhaps the most significant force. Through a combination of dominance in numbers, increased purchasing power, wider dissemination of knowledge, democratic expression, and legislative change, 'the masses' are rising up again, this time in peaceful, evolutionary change and are demanding greater control of their lives, and a greater say in all aspects of our society.

Royalty and clergy relied on their almost unquestioned status to achieve control of the other major determinants of power: strength, money, and knowledge. For the professional classes, it has been through knowledge that money, status, and strength – both political and legislative – were achieved. However, in the last two decades, the professional classes have found that their own almost unquestioned monopoly, on knowledge, so crucial to their power, is being eroded, and, through this change, that their 'right' to the other determinants, and rewards of power, is also being challenged.

Information has become more readily available than ever before. The old adage of 'knowledge is power' remains valid; ordinary citizens want more of both: knowledge and power. Politicians know this, and know too that citizens are voters. Therefore, we have seen a range of government policies based on 'transparency' and 'choice' – the publication of league tables (for schools, hospitals, even police forces), and the reports of an increasing host of 'inspection bodies', covering all manner of public services, and there have been promises of more, from all political parties.

At the same time, we have seen the rise of an even more powerful means of disseminating information and of widening the reach of the ordinary citizen: the Internet. This is a force that many governments, although professing to 'transparency', actually fear, as it is less amenable to the means of control that governments deploy: what to release, how, when, and where.

Therefore, while the French national anthem – 'le Marseillaise', the battle hymn of the revolution – exhorts citizens to rise up, as their time has come, it may be that that was a promise deferred, that only now may be fulfilled.

Empowered citizens; empowered consumers

Now it is governments, rather than revolutionary leaders, that advocate, albeit within carefully defined areas, a more empowered citizenry. We all have become familiar with a new type of citizen, who tends to better educated, is more prosperous, has improved access to information, certainly has higher expectations, and is less deferential to authority and to the traditional class structures. Furthermore, aspirations have changed; no longer does the citizenry contemplate revolution, instead it seeks a contented life, and consumer goods and experiences to support this.

This new 'Consumerist' agenda can be summarized as quantity, quality, deregulation, and accountability. In a less polite analysis, as 'I want it, I want it to be good, I don't mind where I get it from, but I'll sue if I'm not happy with it'. Before you dismiss this as excessive stereotyping, what went through your mind when you last bought a computer, or a car?

Although these 'assertive citizens' may still be in the minority, their numbers are rising, their power is increasing, and they are being encouraged by government policies. Although there undoubtedly are problems with the government's 'choice' policies, they do cater to this particular type of voter and are intended to be a driver of economic and social change.

Empowered citizens; empowered patients

Doctors tend to deplore any description of the care they provide for patients as a service to consumers. However, health economists and politicians do not, and they are driving these changes. In terms of the economics and the politics, the advantages are clear: consumers like to feel they have greater control, and consumers are voters. Furthermore, what a bonus, if, through the empowerment of patients, the power of the medical profession is reduced.

Although there may only be a small number of patients who arrive in your clinic with many pages printed out from the Internet, having chosen and booked their appointment time, wanting to discuss with you, in detail, the full implications of the treatment options you are suggesting, all indications are that they are the vanguard of a much wider social trend.

However, this great wave of consumerism that appears to be threatening to wash away the world of the professionals, may not be as threatening as this initial analysis may suggest. Indeed, as will be shown in the following sections, it may be that by adapting our professionalism, more fully to work with the patients and society we serve, doctors will be able to respond more appropriately to the dramatically changing needs of this new century. These changes may also provide the basis for a new relationship between the medical profession and society: a renewed 'social contract'.

More empowered during the delivery of health care

The primacy of the autonomy of the patient is one of the key concepts of modern medical ethics; it is also a key factor of patient empowerment. If each individual is recognized as autonomous and has the capacity to make decisions regarding their health care, then the acknowledgement of this by the doctor(s) looking after them will encourage the development of a relationship based on partnership rather than paternalism.

It is acknowledged that much work has yet to be done to ensure that those concepts are fully embedded in the delivery of health care, by doctors and by patients. Although some patients, and indeed some doctors, appear to prefer a model of (hopefully) benign paternalism, the overall trend is clear, with the 'great institutions' of the medical profession making clear their commitment to this re-balancing of the patient–doctor relationship.

Many claims are made for increasing the empowerment of patients, some of which are even based on valid evidence. However, some claims appear to be an excuse for other, more political changes. It is evident that a greater sense of autonomy and empowerment does provide for improved patient experience, a result both confirmed, and encouraged by surveys of patients. There also is evidence that suggests that patients are more likely to be compliant with therapy if they have a greater sense of involvement in the decision-making regarding their treatment.

Patient empowerment also has been linked with improved outcomes for patients, but there is debate as to whether these results are owing to factors such as improved compliance, or bias owing to the improved education, socio-economic status of more empowered patients, or other factors. Similar issues apply when patient empowerment is linked to greater awareness about health, which is more likely among more educated patients. This also runs counter to one of the claims made for greater patient empowerment, that this will reduce health inequalities.

One rapidly enters the area of political debate when one recognizes that more empowered patients, who are more able to be involved in decision-making regarding their health care, may also wish to exert choice as to when, where, and even how their health care is delivered. Such matters are at the heart of the 'choice agenda' for patients in the NHS – which wishes to encourage change – and frequently are cited as a reason in the United States for resisting change to their health care system.

Common to both agendas is the wish to focus the service more fully on those it serves and, through giving patients greater rights and responsibilities, thereby to ensure that the service functions more efficiently and effectively. However, in the United Kingdom this is seen as a means of achieving politically desired reconfiguration of the health service, which inevitably would result from patients asserting their choice to go where they feel they would be better cared for. With greater information on hospitals now available, and patients apparently more able to 'choose and book', the foundations of this scenario already have been prepared.

Patient and doctor

For centuries the relationship between patient and doctor was characterized by benign paternalism: the patient deferred to the wise doctor to diagnose his or her malady and decide how best to deal with this; in return, (almost always) the doctor was afforded status and wealth. This relationship was based primarily on the near-monopoly of knowledge held by the medical profession.

In the last two decades, information on the human body, the ills that afflict it, and the means of treating those has become widely available. Over a similar period, whether by a causal relationship or otherwise, society has become less deferential. The relationship between patient and doctor has changed and will change further.

A new relationship is being developed, where the critical factor is the sharing of information: by the patient and by his or her doctor(s). This reflects greater emphasis on the primacy of autonomy of the individual and a model where medical decision-making is shared, and where good communication, in both directions, is essential. Patients and doctors work together to deal with medical problems, and the results of tests and letters between doctors are shared with the patient. Patients are encouraged to seek relevant information – from information leaflets, telephone helplines, and relevant websites – and, particularly if they have a chronic condition, to join a 'disease care' group. New alliances are being developed between patients and doctors, patients and other patients, patients and their carers.

More empowered in the quality of health care

Patients also are becoming more active in aspects of health care that go beyond their conventional involvement; most notably, in the areas of quality of care. Using an analysis based on quality improvement, assurance, and control, it is possible to review how extensive that involvement has become.

Examples of how patients, and other lay people have become more empowered in improving quality include the employment of 'simulated patients' in the training of students and junior doctors, and even having patients as teachers. In both cases, patients are able to bring their personal experience to the learning process. Patients and their carers may become active in patient liaison groups, often working with doctors to lobby for better care. The GMC routinely consults widely regarding its guidance and receives many responses from individuals and from patients' groups; this good practice is being followed by some medical schools that consult on the details of their undergraduate syllabus. Another area is that of research, a particularly sensitive area, where medical opinion and public opinion sometimes are not aligned; by having lay members of ethics committees these concerns usually can be addressed.

Because doctors have become more accountable for the quality of care they provide, patients have become more empowered in assuring that quality. For some years, many specialities have encouraged patients to complete surveys and contribute to the audit of the service provided; now, the NHS has national patient surveys, which allow trusts to be compared, and specific issues to be monitored. The NHS complaints procedures have been extensively revised to ensure that complaints from patients or their families receive necessary attention, are responded to within a defined timescale and, where appropriate, provide an opportunity for improving the service. For individual doctors, it is likely that multi-source feedback will be a key component of revalidation; in most specialities that will include responses from patients. Patients, or their lay representatives, also are becoming involved in the increasingly rigorous inspections that all hospitals and general practice premises are required to fulfil.

One of the more controversial areas being considered is whether patients should have the right to be able to access their doctor's performance data.

This already is the case for some specialities in some countries and, in the United Kingdom, such figures are published for cardiac surgery. There are concerns regarding the need to address, through statistical correction, differences in case complexity, and worries that a simplistic presentation of what is complex information may lead to inappropriate conclusions. The 'law of unintended consequences' also must be considered; although it has been suggested that doctors might alter their treatment criteria to reduce the likelihood of poor patient outcomes affecting their figures, it is encouraging to note that early data do not indicate that this is occurring.

Since the 1970s there has also been an increasing involvement of lay people in the regulation of medicine; in the most clear numerical terms, on the Council of the GMC, the proportion of lay members has risen from 15% to 50%. This reflects a change for all professional regulatory bodies in the United Kingdom, many of which now have a majority of lay council members. In the case of the GMC, this has led to much debate as to what form of regulation doctors now have, with terms such as 'professionally led' and 'co-regulation' being suggested; there is no debate, however, over the demise of 'self-regulation'.

These numerical changes, while dramatic, have been small compared with the changes in policy that have occurred, much of that within the last decade. There has been a shift from the old model of regulation, that could be characterized as 'thou shalt not', to a more balanced approach, in which 'thou shalt' is considered as important, if not more important. Accompanying this change in regulatory 'philosophy' has been progress towards revalidation, that follows from the decision that all doctors, on a regular basis, must be able to demonstrate their continuing fitness to practise. The obvious consequence of these profound changes is that doctors will be more accountable than ever; a requirement strongly supported by patients, lay people, the media, and politicians.

These groups also have demanded changes in the area of fitness to practice hearings. When compared with the number of practising doctors, and the number of patients they care for, the number of such cases is small. However, the nature of these cases means that they receive a disproportionate amount of attention in the media and, despite the statutory independence of the GMC, intervention from some politicians. In a shift that will affect all health care professions, no longer will all such cases be considered according to a standard of proof 'beyond reasonable doubt' but rather, in many cases, 'on balance of probabilities'. Although it is unlikely that this will be the last word on this subject – European law may provide a means of challenge – these changes were introduced following pressure from outside the medical profession: 'self-regulation' certainly is no more.

Although the increasing involvement of patients and other lay people in all aspects of the quality of health care may appear threatening to some doctors, this represents a shift that more accurately reflects the primary duty of a doctor: to make the care of their patient their first concern. When patients are saying that they want a more balanced relationship, in which they are more involved in determining the care that they receive, the medical profession must recognize the need for change. In the United Kingdom, to a large extent, despite this having been an uncomfortable process for the medical profession, this has indeed been the case, and considerable change has been achieved.

More empowered in health care politics

Successive governments have encouraged patients and the public to have a greater say in the planning, commissioning, and delivery of health care. At an individual level, these forms of advocacy include patients, particularly those with long-term conditions, being provided greater information from their doctor(s) on how to be more involved in determining their care. Another example is that of Patient Advisory Liaison Services that assist patients and their carers in finding their way around the complex networks of hospital services.

As part of the shift towards greater responsiveness towards local needs, for those hospitals that have become foundation trusts, members of the public are encouraged to contribute to decision-making. All parts of the primary care and hospital sectors are required to consult the population they serve more fully than ever before. Although some may feel that these are just small steps, inadequately followed, these small steps are on a path not yet walked by the NHS and are likely to lead to a much larger road.

One of the reasons for this is the extent to which the media, both local and national, have become involved in health care. There are, as always, the usual stories – scandals, problems, miraculous cures – but now there also are articles about how well the local hospital is doing, as compared with other hospitals, and what patients can do to demand better services.

Patients are being encouraged to become organized, to advocate for better quality care, for care that is focused on their needs rather than on the needs of health care providers. This works for individual patients, some of whom have even taken legal action to ensure that they receive certain medication, or reimbursement for treatment abroad. It also works for groups of patients; patient representative groups, frequently organized around a particular medical condition, have become adept at political lobbying, locally, nationally, and in Europe.

This greater voice for patients has an impact far greater than merely affecting the provision of local services. When a relative challenges the prime minister about inadequate care, it hits the headlines; when a legal challenge has multi-million pound implications for the NHS budget, the politicians listen. Politicians know that, aside from all else, patients, their relatives, the public, are voters.

The implications for the medical profession

These changes, although individually apparently small, collectively are having a profound impact on the relationships between patients and their doctor(s), and between the medical profession and society as a whole.

The greatest changes relate to the increased sharing of information by doctors with their patients and, with that, the recognition that patients will become more involved in decision-making regarding their care. Although most doctors have adapted their consultation style to recognize these patient preferences, these issues are detailed in the GMC document on consent, which provides guidance on the manner in which doctors are expected to communicate with their patients regarding clinical decisions. The 'partnership model' that this requires involves improved, two-way communication, in which the patient's wishes regarding their care are more fully acknowledged, and the doctor is expected to provide guidance, rather than direction, through a range of treatment options. This model also has implications for patients who will have the opportunity, not merely to assert their rights but also to take greater responsibility for their health care, and for the decisions that they make regarding this. For it to work effectively, the 'partnership model' requires both parties, doctor and patient, to commit to a professional relationship based on trust, the sharing of all relevant information, and greater consideration of what, among available options, would be the most appropriate health care intervention(s) for the patient as an individual.

Although these changes require doctors and patients to adapt to a new professional relationship, there also are implications for the relationship between individual patients and the NHS as a whole. As has occurred in all countries, owing to factors such as demographic changes, and the greater available of more complex forms of treatment, the overall cost of health care in the United Kingdom has increased considerably. Another factor fuelling this rise in costs has been the increase in patients' expectations. As a result, there have been legal cases in which the individual patient's need for medical resources has been tested against society's requirement, in a health system that has considerable, but limited resources, to determine the allocation of those resources. These cases have tested what alternatively are described as priority-setting or rationing, at both local and national levels, raising the question of who should manage need in the health care system: patients, professionals, or politicians?

The implications for the medical profession of such questions, and of the changes that have led to these events, are considerable. The interface between the health care needs of individual patients, and medical ethics, and the law of the land, has brought into focus the extent to which patients can demand health care services, to which doctors can make decisions, based on their professional judgement, of whether certain treatments can be clinically justified, and to which the NHS is responsible for funding care. It has also raised concerns as to whether patients should take greater responsibility for their lifestyle choices.

Creating the future

Although discussion, debate, and legal challenge on these matters likely will continue for many years, as has been shown above, the larger reality is that these changes are part of an unstoppable 'great wave' of social change. Accordingly, rather than attempting to resist change, the challenge to the medical profession should be how best to harness for good effect the energy of this wave of change.

By virtue of their professional relationship – based on trust between a person seeking care and the professional from whom they receive that care – there is a natural alliance between patients and doctors that, if developed, could form the basis for a renewed contract between society and the medical profession. Rather than this relationship being seen as a zero-sum negotiation, in which patients and society 'win', and doctors and the medical profession 'lose', there is the potential for a new 'social contract' to develop, in which doctors – who derive their empowerment from patients and society – re-establish that contract, based on agreed greater empowerment for patients. This mutualism of empowerment in the relationship between patients and doctors could also provide the basis for the mutual agenda, of society and the medical profession, to advocate for improved healthcare and greater resources for the NHS.

A new professionalism

To achieve this new 'social contract' it will be necessary for the medical profession to refresh its model of what it means to be a doctor. Such a change would be akin to the changes that have occurred in the medical profession in response to other historic changes in society. The following characterization is merely a convenient summary: in the 'age of kings and clergy', doctors were 'magician healers', treating according to traditional knowledge, based on trial and error; following the 'great wave' of enlightenments and revolutions that occurred in many human cultures, doctors incorporated the rapid expansion of knowledge and experimental method to become 'scientist carers', practising in accordance with the values and needs of the 'age of the professionals'.

The 'great wave' of consumerism already has produced enormous social changes that have affected all of us as citizens: greater information, greater purchasing opportunity, and greater power as citizens. Harnessed appropriately, it could also support the creation of a new medical professionalism. In our modern age, the 'age of the consumer', the challenge to doctors is to adapt again, to become 'practitioner guides': practising in partnership with the patient, analysing all available information, considering a wider range of management options, working with expanded and changing health care teams, performing clinical interventions that likely will become increasingly complex and specialized, and being more accountable for their professional performance and their continuing fitness to practise.

References

General Medical Council. (2007). *Good Medical Practice*. London: General Medical Council.

General Medical Council. (2008). *Consent: Patients and Doctors Making Decisions Together*. London: General Medical Council.

Chapter 17

Psychiatric ethics and the 'new professionalism'

Michael Robertson and Garry Walter

Introduction

Since the 1980s, health care has evolved into a huge enterprise that represents a significant expenditure by government and private sectors. As such, the medical profession has become a component of an industry in which issues of public policy, market forces, and consumer demands are key influences. Within this altered context, the nature of professionalism has changed, as have the ethical concerns physicians face. Traditional notions of profe
ssional ethics have evolved from a focus on the doctor–patient relationship, through the Hippocratic tradition and later in the contributions of Percival (1985) and Ross (1939).

The 'new professionalism' refers to the evolution of medical ethics in light of a number of changes in health care, including the scale of health care; the rise of interdisciplinary health care and prominence of the biopsychosocial model in mental health, technical progress, increased literacy about health care in the community, public policy and expectations of third parties.

In this chapter, we take the position that the profession of psychiatry has negotiated this change by adopting an ethical approach that is best considered a form of social contract. In this social contract, psychiatrists are engaged in a three-way relationship that includes their patients and the other stakeholders in health care. The ethical dilemmas faced by psychiatrists in such a context are those that emerge out of the tension between responsibilities to patients and to third parties. We argue that these ethical dilemmas are most evident in circumstances where the social contract fails.

What is the 'new' professionalism?

The *Oxford English Dictionary* (1993) defines a profession as follows:

> An occupation whose core element is work, based on the mastery of a complex body of knowledge and skills. It is a vocation in which knowledge of some department of

science or learning, or the practice of an art founded on it, is used in the service of others. Its members profess a commitment to competence, integrity, morality, altruism, and *the promotion of the public good within their domain*. These commitments form the basis of a *social contract between a profession and society*, which in return grants the profession autonomy in practice and the privilege of self-regulation. Professions and their members are accountable to those served and to society (our italics).

The key elements of this definition appear to be the existence of a contract of sorts between a professional group (or individual professional) and society, the promotion of public good, and a number of desirable personal qualities or 'virtues'. In exchange, the group is accorded professional autonomy and the capacity to self-regulate (Cruess & Cruess, 1997).

The original Hippocratic tradition was *primum non nocere* (first, do no harm). This holds that any action of a physician must benefit, and in no way harm, the patient. The situation has changed and the Hippocratic tradition in medical ethics has waned (Pellegrino, 1993) owing to the presumed effect of the evolution of Western societies into consumer economies (Cruess, Johnston, & Cruess, 2002), the commercialization of the health system and technological advances in medicine (Cruess et al., 2002; Dyer, 1988). It has been argued that, in light of such developments, the craft of medicine has been transformed into a service industry in which technical skills are traded in a market place. As such, the notions of 'physicianly' virtue and the Hippocratic tradition have been lost. The scale of the practice of medicine has also increased exponentially. In developed countries, medicine has changed in one or two generations from a 'cottage industry' to one consuming a significant portion of a country's gross domestic product (Cruess et al., 2002).

Professional ethics, arguably, have three core components – specialized training and the acquisition of specialized skills; the provision of expert assistance to those in need and vulnerable; and the virtues of trustworthiness, efficacy, and knowledge that ultimately enhance the common good and aggregate well-being (Fullinwider, 1996). A profession is, therefore, a group that possess specialized skills and knowledge applied for a collective good (ABIM Foundation, ACP-ASIM Foundation & EFIM, 2002; Pellegrino, 1999).

Several physicians' organizations have jointly outlined a series of principles and responsibilities for the medical profession, which integrate the recent influences on medical practice (ABIM Foundation, ACP-ASIM Foundation & EFIM, 2002). In this new code, the principles of patient welfare, patient autonomy, and social justice are juxtaposed with the responsibilities of commitment to professional competence, honesty with patients, confidentiality, appropriate relations, improving quality of care, improving access to care, ensuring a fair distribution of finite resources, pursuit of scientific knowledge, and maintenance of trust by managing conflicts of interest and professional responsibilities.

Such aspirational statements have the two themes of physicians possessing of a set of desirable virtues and the role of advocacy. These highlight the values of the medical profession. A recent study of Australian psychiatrists (Robertson, Kerridge, & Walter, 2009) suggested that the main values in their work were the value of the patient, the value of sophisticated understanding, the value of reflection, and the value of advocacy. These values are well represented in professional codes of ethics.

Professional ethical autonomy is therefore given on the understanding that professionals will devote themselves to serving the best interests of society and will self-regulate to maintain high quality care and beneficent conduct (Cruess & Cruess, 1997). The tenets of this beneficent conduct have been specified as patient welfare and autonomy as well as the just allocation of resources (ABIM Foundation, ACP-ASIM Foundation & EFIM, 2002).

One of the key elements in this definition of professionalism is the 'contract' between the profession and society, in particular what is defined as a 'collective good'. This collective aspect of professionalism is balanced with the Hippocratic tradition of the individual physician as non-maleficent healer. There is potential for significant tension between these two traditions of 'ethics' as it is possible that an expected action in the interests of a collective good may be deleterious to an individual patient.

The tension between these potentially conflicting roles creates a degree of anxiety about the profession of medicine (Cruess et al. 2002). As Cruess and others have argued, these anxieties have led to a reflection upon the values that have traditionally characterized medicine.

An additional complexity in this mix is provided by the involvement of third parties, a recent phenomenon in the history of medicine brought about by market forces. Such a dilemma has been outlined specifically in the case of psychiatry, with a call to reflect upon the inherent tensions within the notion of medicine as the trade of applied technical skills (Dyer, 1988).

In any setting, the psychiatric profession is thoroughly integrated with the norms of the society in which it exists. Such norms influence both diagnostic and treatment approaches, and exert coercive pressure upon psychiatrists through the imposition of laws that govern many aspects of the way they practise their craft. As such, there is a particularity to the ethics of psychiatry functioning in different sociocultural settings. Such an intricate network of relationships and obligations implores psychiatrists to consider the integration of their personal sense of an ethical life and the virtues of a physician, the discourses of professional ethics of the psychiatric profession, and the expectations of the social contract, clearly embodied in law.

It has been argued, therefore, that psychiatric ethics are a network of interactions between the individual morality of the psychiatrist, the immediate collegiate relationships of the psychiatrist, and the relationship between the psychiatric profession and the broader society (Robertson & Walter, 2007).

The social contract and professional ethics in psychiatry

The critical issue in professional ethics and its related dilemmas in psychiatry is that of the social contract. In this section, we will outline the tenets of this approach to moral philosophy in the light of two critical thinkers in the field – Hobbes and Rawls.

Hobbes (1651/1985) postulated that humans were, by nature, prone to act in self-interest. In Hobbes' view, society would deteriorate to a violent state of anarchy unless regulated by laws. In essence, all members of society would act out of their self-interest to participate in an agreement in which a set of laws would create a society where no one was allowed to act in an exploitative or violent manner. Hobbes proposed that a powerful sovereign (or 'Leviathan') would enforce the social contract arrangement by punishing or excluding those persons who violated the social contract arrangement. Applied to a professional context, the contractarian approach to ethics involves the assumption that a professional group will, primarily out of self-interest, abide by an agreed set of expectations of behaviour and conduct. This is usually in exchange for a level of professional autonomy or self-regulation. When a profession is seen to fail in this agreement, in either a specific instance or an overall manner, society tends to respond through enacting legislation to enforce a particular change. For example, if there are a number of instances of failure of a professional group to maintain standards of practice, then a society's legislators will enact laws to force the profession to introduce such standards. In essence, the penalty for a profession's failing to meet the expectations of the social contract is the loss of various components of self-regulation.

The social contract tradition in medical ethics is problematic in the setting of psychiatry. Society may encourage certain expectations of the psychiatric profession, which are to the detriment of people with mental illness. This places the psychiatric profession in a position of conflict between obligation to a patient and to the society in the professional social contract. The clearest example of this relates to public safety. After the rare instance of a person suffering a mental illness harming another person, society may, through its legislators or its institutions, emphasize the expectation that psychiatrists must manage risk more effectively. Putting aside the obvious limits of this as an undertaking, this may result in the psychiatric profession being expected to act more coercively in the treatment of people with mental illness to protect the public rather than provide care for patients. This highlights the fundamental dilemma in the social contract tradition of ethics applied to a professional group, where the presumed 'common good' of society comes into conflict with the interests of the patient.

John Rawls (1971, 1993, 2001) developed a conception of distributive justice over his career. His notion of the social contract considered more specifically the just allocation of limited resources within a 'well-ordered society'. Rawls saw that all members of a 'well-ordered society' had equal entitlement to access social goods in order to have the opportunity of living fulfilling lives. He took the Kantian view that individual fulfilment is a product of autonomy or rational self-governance. As such, social goods are instrumental in achieving this, and the just distribution of these social goods assists members of society to achieve this autonomous existence. As Nussbaum points out, such an approach falters when we consider the situation of those whose capacity for autonomy is impaired life-long. A person with disabling chronic schizophrenia may never be truly capable of autonomy and so their needs are poorly met in Rawls' philosophy. As such, Nussbaum builds on the so-called capabilities approach to justice (Sen, 1993) to provide a more workable account of the primary social goods at the centre of Rawls' distributive justice (Nussbaum, 1999). Nussbaum's concept of 'capabilities' defined these as the necessary preconditions for a person's capacity to flourish through aspiring to a life characterized by dignity. This is in contrast to Rawls' conception of a life's goal of realizing Kantian autonomy. The capabilities extend from reasonable life expectancy, and sensory and bodily integrity, through to capacity for affiliative behaviour, play, and some control over one's environment. Nussbaum thus sees that the ends of just public policy with regard to people with psychiatric or intellectual disabilities is the guarantee of their basic dignity (Nussbaum, 2006).

Rawls' theories have been extended to the specific areas of health care by Norman Daniels (Daniels, 1995). Daniels defines 'health care' broadly, as encompassing individual medical services, preventative interventions, public health initiatives, workplace safety, and social resources for chronically ill and disabled. Daniels argues that the 'right' to health care carries the implicit assumption that access to health care is on par with other civil rights, which equates health care with other social goods.

The rationale of providing health care paid for by third parties, such as government, is, therefore, to help restore normal function by decreasing the effect of disease or disability. This compensates for the 'natural lottery' in which liability for disease is considered an accident of birth, rather than the individual failings of the sufferer. A guarantee of access to health care does not have the goal to enhance well-being or general capability but merely correcting for the natural lottery.

Sabin and Daniels have applied these concepts specifically to mental health (Sabin & Daniels, 1994). They advance a 'normal function model' in light of how mental illness may affect that function. They propose that the goal of mental health care is to obviate the disadvantage arising from mental illness, thus making everyone equal competitors for social resources. Their model of justice, achieved through mental health care, has three dimensions:

1. A 'normal function model' of mental health care seeking to create 'normal' competitors for social resources.
2. A 'capability model' seeking to create equal competitors for resources.
3. A 'welfare model' addressing the fact that people suffer because of attitudes or behaviours they did not choose and cannot choose to overcome, which should justify access to mental health care

The 'normal function' model allows a society to draw a plausible boundary around the scope for insurance coverage. Sabin and Daniels argue that the capability and the welfare models are the most morally substantive but are the most problematic in implementation.

Thus, on two fronts of the social contract, the psychiatric profession confronts ethical dilemmas – those related to just allocation of resources and those related to acting out of self-interest to maintain this contractarian relationship. In both instances, there is potential for these imperatives to come into conflict with the values of psychiatrists, in particular those surrounding their relationship with particular patients. We will return to this issue at the end of the chapter.

The relationship between societal and psychiatric values

In considering a contract between the psychiatric profession and the community, it is necessary to consider the values of both groups. If the conduct of the psychiatric profession within such a contract sees a clash of values, this will lead to ethical dilemmas in the profession. There has been little empirical investigation into the values of the psychiatric profession (Borry, Schotsmans, & Dierickx, 2008); other than induct from the codes of ethics of different national or international organizations of psychiatrists, this awaits further research.

Even more problematic is identifying a set of values held by a community. The philosopher Bernard Gert coined the term 'common morality theory'. The common morality reflects the broad values of citizens living in a stable democratic society (Gert, 1998, 2004). Such values can be considered descriptive as they reflect what people actually do in different situations. According to Gert, his normative moral system is based upon five basic harms – death, pain, disability, loss of freedom, and loss of pleasure. From these five harms, Gert derives 10 moral rules reflecting the common morality of a society:

1. Do not kill.
2. Do not cause pain.
3. Do not disable.
4. Do not deprive of freedom.
5. Do not deprive of pleasure.
6. Do not deceive.
7. Keep your promises.
8. Do not cheat.
9. Obey the law.
10. Do your duty.

The first five of these rules prohibit inflicting the five basic harms directly, whereas the second five prohibit actions that may cause the same harms indirectly. These 10 moral rules are not absolute in that their violations are not always wrong.

Gert justified his philosophy by arguing that every rational agent will ultimately endorse adopting a moral system that required everyone to act morally in regard to other moral agents. The basic harms would be seen to be almost universalizable in that all rational people would agree that these are the basic values of stable societies. Gert calls this 'the blindfold of justice' in that these rules are independent of religious, nationalistic, or scientific beliefs. In collaboration with K. Danner Clouser, Gert proposed that medical ethics is little more than an application of common morality to specific medical ethical dilemmas (Clouser, 1970, 1973, 1995; Clouser & Gert, 1990).

The approach of common morality appears to represent the basic tenets of the kind of social contract envisioned by Hobbes. Its injunctions aspire to little more than avoidance of criminal activity. The values evident in the common morality seem to indicate the basic goods of a functioning society and most likely indicate the kind of consensus that 'moral strangers' (Engelhardt, 1996), that is, members of society from diverse backgrounds would be able to negotiate.

From the perspective of stable liberal democracies, the notion of common morality presents a plausible foundation of the values of a society. In the context of a globalized psychiatric profession (see below), the question is raised of how international organizations of psychiatric professionals respond to societies where capital punishment or restrictions of human rights are practised. This invites the notion of moral relativism, which contends that the values of particular groups can only be understood from within their specific context. This 'vulgar moral relativism' (Williams, 1972) is problematic in that it invites the 'anything goes approach', which is anathema to many psychiatrists in the liberal West. The position of 'sophisticated moral relativism' (Wong, 1991) offers a better approach. In such a consideration of the customs of different groups, the sophisticated moral relativist approach considers the efficacy of a society or culture's mores and customs in guaranteeing the kind of social goods consistent with a social contract. Rather than tolerate the excesses of a ruthless tyrant in a failed state, the sophisticated approach to moral relativism considers how capital punishment or involuntary detention is relevant to the success of a particular society.

Changes in psychiatric practice

Foucault (1965) had argued that the conceptualization of madness and psychiatry was contextual to the society in which it occurred. By extension, changes in the psychiatric profession parallel changes in society and culture. The history of psychiatry in the West has seen the end of the asylum era and the rise of notions of 'mental health' and the empowerment of those affected by mental illness. The three main influences on the professional ethics of psychiatry are sociocultural, political, and technological.

The process of change in the psychiatric profession paralleled similar changes in society's approach to mental illness. The concept of alienism was abandoned for those of 'mental hygiene' and ultimately 'mental health' (Ridenour, 1961). The emergence of the mental health paradigm placed the care of mentally ill people in the broad context of the social and cultural determinants of mental health and mental illness. One of the main assumptions of the mental health movement was that the prevention of mental illness should be a focus of public policy. As such, psychiatry became one component of a social process that aspired to diminish the impact of mental illness on a community. In the 1980s, the emergence of Engel's biopsychosocial approach (Engel, 1977, 1980) exerted a significant influence on the way in which mental health services operated. Psychiatry was practised in a multidisciplinary environment and the biomedical discourse of mental illness became a more pluralistic one (Ghaemi, 2003).

Political interests have become increasingly prominent influences in the ethical dilemmas faced by the psychiatric profession. In 'new world' countries, psychiatry had a prominent role in influencing immigration policies, and therefore the composition of these new societies. The association of mental illness, criminality, and immigrants were important themes in the history of Australian (Dax, 1981) and Argentine psychiatry (Plotkin, 2001) in the early twentieth century. The potentially malignant influence of politics on the psychiatric profession found one of its most disturbing manifestations in the crimes of the psychiatric profession in the Union of Soviet Socialist Republics, where many psychiatrists colluded with the use of psychiatric diagnosis and treatment to suppress political dissent. The Soviet psychiatric example highlights one of the main dilemmas in the contractarian approach to professional ethics in psychiatry – what ought psychiatrists do when the State is prosecuting an immoral agenda?

Although by no means morally equivalent with the Soviet experience, the recent debates in the United Kingdom over the proposed 'Dangerous Severe Personality Disorder' (Appelbaum, 2005) legislation provide an example of the troubled relationship between the psychiatric profession, party politics, and social expectations. The proposed laws would enable preventative detention of potentially dangerous individuals, 'diagnosed' with psychopathic or personality disorders, in secure psychiatric hospitals. Such laws arise in the context of public concern over the association of violent crime and personality disorder, and the populist political response to such sentiment. Indeed, in the United Kingdom it has been argued that the psychiatric profession has been 'held hostage to the fortunes of knee-jerk UK government responses to generally ill-informed, and often hostile, public opinion' and therefore 'conditioned to the threat of public backlash and professional criticism' (Welsh & Deahl, 2002). Both the Soviet and British examples highlight a distinct set of professional ethical dilemmas occurring in the setting of political interests. In such contexts, professional ethics in psychiatry confront the most basic concerns of human rights.

Progress in the neurosciences has also influenced the ethical dilemmas faced by psychiatrists. The discovery of the antipsychotic properties of chlorpromazine in 1952 heralded the prospect of those patients suffering schizophrenia, who had been incapable of independent living, residing in the community. In the face of this, aspirations to community-based psychiatric care evolved. The reality has been more one of the mentally ill facing severe social disadvantage, lack of access to care, and prisons becoming de facto psychiatric hospitals (White & Whiteford, 2006) – the prevalence of psychiatric disorder is significantly higher in the prison population than the community (Butler et al., 2006). In the 1960s, the global trend to community care led to a process of deinstitutionalization in Australia (Lewis, 1988) although the process resulted in those suffering mental illness being 'removed from one form of incarceration only to end up in another' (Coleborne, 2003). The period from the 1960s saw significant levels of divestment of government in community mental health services and the defaulting of many services to poorly funded non-government organizations (Mental Health Council of Australia, 2005).

Further paradoxes emerged from the technological progress that confronted psychiatry. In July 1990, US President George HW Bush issued 'presidential proclamation 6158' deeming the 1990s the 'decade of the brain' (DOB). Although the anticipated flourishing in neuroscience held promise, even the most sanguine of assessments of the DOB could only offer further anticipation of ultimate clinical utility:

> Even when a cure or effective treatment does not yet exist – the attention attracted by recent breakthroughs ... has induced a clear expectation that treatments are not too far away.
>
> (Jones & Mendell, 1999)

Regardless of actual progress, the DOB did facilitate the transformation of psychiatry into an enterprise focused upon the neurosciences. One of the concomitants of the emergence of this biological psychiatry has been the change in the relationship between the psychiatric profession and commercial interests. The most notable of these is the pharmaceutical industry. The discovery of the antidepressant properties of the anti-tuberculosis drug iproniazad initiated a process of research into the potential for clinically and commercially successful antidepressant compounds (Healy, 1997) – some have argued that the diagnosis of depression has expanded in response to the commercial development of antidepressant medications (Healy, 2004). The relationship between psychiatry, and medical profession generally, and the pharmaceutical industry has been the subject of debate within the profession (Wazana & Primeau, 2002) and within the community (Angell, 2009). The relationship between the psychiatric profession and the pharmaceutical industry has been of concern in the influence of the latter on academic (Healy & Thase, 2003) and professional activities (Green, 2008).

The other factor influencing the professional landscape in psychiatry has been the emergence of a form of globalized psychiatry. The foundation of the World Psychiatric Association and its ethical proclamations in the wake of the crimes of Soviet psychiatrists (1978) avers that the psychiatric profession is a global enterprise that shares a common set of values enshrined in proclamations such as the Declaration of Madrid (1997). Moreover, the effect of commercially successful classification systems such as the *American Psychiatric Association's Diagnostic and Statistical Manual of Mental Disorders* has been the adoption of an approach to the classification of psychiatric disorders that has transcended cultures and created a de facto globalization of the psychiatric profession (Kirk & Kutchins, 1992, 1997).

Psychiatry and social justice

Throughout this chapter, we have argued that the professional ethical dilemmas surrounding psychiatry are best considered in the context of social contract theory. This does not diminish the importance of other approaches to psychiatric ethics such as virtue or care ethics, but rather provides a model in which psychiatrists can deliberate on the moral quandaries they face as professionals. The successful operation of the social contract involves rational choosers abdicating certain natural rights in exchange for social goods.

There are, however, circumstances where the social contract process appears to fail:

1. What of the mentally ill who may be incapable of rational agreement to the social contract process, yet need the protection of the sovereign?
2. What of those members of society who are 'second class citizens' and do not benefit from the social contract, yet are expected to abide by it?
3. What if the sovereign fails in its responsibilities in enforcing the social contract?

These three scenarios represent manifestations of the 'dual role dilemma' in psychiatry, in that they frequently present quandaries, which place individual psychiatrists, and the profession, in a conflicted position. The essence of this conflict is the responsibility to the individual patient versus to society or the community (Robertson & Walter, 2008). Where there are conflicting imperatives over questions of public safety, as against, an individual patient's right to confidentiality in Tarasoff-; like circumstances (where exists a duty to inform in the case of immediate threat of harm; California. Supreme Court, 1973), the tension tends to resolve in favour of public safety.

In contrast to the so-called moral free-rider, who seeks to benefit from the social contract without abiding by its requirements, those who cannot necessarily commit to the social contract, by virtue of irrationality or impairment, present an ethical dilemma. Most civilized societies provide some form of decent minimum in terms of basic social goods, such as welfare and some access to health care. However, it is apparent that the mentally ill of most developed societies have failed to benefit from the alleged prosperity of the post-industrial globalized economy. Whether this failure to benefit relates to the incapacity of many mentally ill people, either individually or as a group, to advocate on behalf of themselves or more to the stigma associated with mental illness is unclear. In such circumstances, there is a compelling argument for advocacy by psychiatrists on behalf of their patients.

Just allocation of limited mental health care resources is a critical issue is psychiatric ethics and forms part of the World Psychiatric Association's *Declaration of Madrid* (1996), which states 'psychiatrists should be aware of and concerned with the equitable allocation of health resources' (WPA, 1996). Several articles in *The Lancet* have also implored psychiatrists to consider issues of just allocation of resources in a global setting as part of their ethical obligations (Dhanda & Narayah, 2007; Herrman & Swartz, 2007).

One of the main questions over the role of psychiatrist's advocacy on behalf of their patients pertains to the limits of such advocacy. Despite broad canvas of social injustice faced by many people who suffer mental illness, most psychiatrists are more concerned about advocating for their individual patients and the immediate ecological aspects relevant to their patient's experience of their illness. Advocacy in this regard addresses the patient's journey through various social institutions, including health systems and other government utilities such as housing or welfare, insurance systems, the courts, prisons, and immigration. In the specific ethical dilemma of the psychiatrist's role in relation to stigma, this presents another problem with the social contract tradition – that of the 'second class citizen'. Second class citizens are, in essence, those members of society who are expected to fulfil the expectations of the social contract, without reasonable expectation of the benefits. Second class citizens may become so either through latent prejudices within a society (often on racial or gender grounds) or through government policy.

If advocacy is a core focus of professional ethics in psychiatry, how far can it go? In most collective groups of psychiatrists, it is apt that there is a divergence of opinion as to the point at which such advocacy becomes inappropriate. The distinction between the advocacy of an psychiatrist as a professional, as against individual citizen, represents a challenge. In an attempt to resolve this, we propose an 'onion skin model' of advocacy by psychiatrists (Figure 17.1). In this model, there is a core of expertise possessed by psychiatrists and therefore actions in this regard are incontrovertibly psychiatric. As one moves to the outer layers of the model, where questions of community attitudes and public policy are situated, the discourse is less psychiatric and more socio-political. In such instances, the uncontested role of a psychiatrist as a member of a professional group lies in informing the public debate over matters of policy and community attitudes and less direct political action. The importance of this model is that the further away one gets from the core business of psychiatry – defined as assessment and treatment of symptoms and impairment – the less substantive is the role of the psychiatrist in advocacy. The true value of this

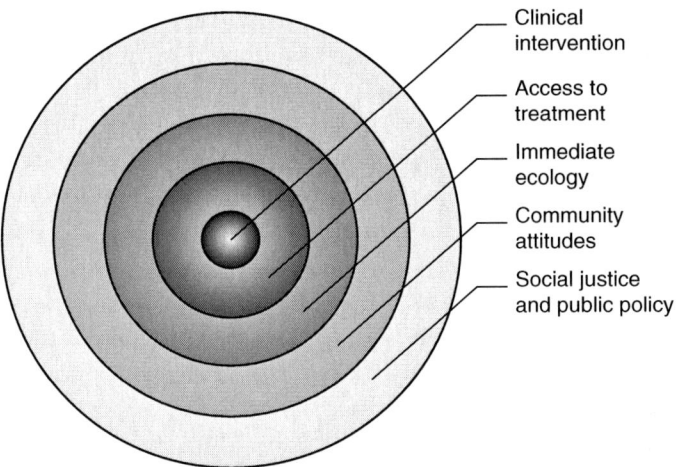

Fig. 17.1 The onion skin model of advocacy and justice

model is that it avoids the either/or approach to advocacy and, more significantly, provides a coherent basis for levels of advocacy, proportionate to a psychiatrist's expertise.

At the core of the model is the advocacy for best treatment for the patient in a clinical setting. This may include peer review or the advocacy among medical colleagues. The next level describes the capacity of patients to access treatment, whether it be medication, inpatient care, or appropriate psychological management. This may involve representations to third parties or institutional bureaucracies. The next layer describes the scope of advocacy for an individual patient in areas such as access to housing, welfare benefits, access to employment or other social goods. This advocacy is often achieved through advising government or non-government agencies of the clinical aspects of a patient's circumstances. This may also involve providing clinical information to civil or criminal courts. Beyond these is the role of advocacy in attempting to influence unhelpful community attitudes, particularly those that involve stigmatizing patients. Increasingly, dedicated non-government agencies have been tasked with this responsibility, resulting in psychiatrists participating in a clinical advisory rather than public advocacy role.

In the United States, the problem of advocacy has been most acute in the face of the implementation of market forces in health care, under the auspices of Managed Care. Managed Care has delivered a number of 'unethical' health systems in the United States, leading to calls for psychiatrists to resist the processes in systems that disadvantage the mentally ill (Green & Bloch, 2001). There is accumulating evidence that managed mental health care may adversely affect clinical outcomes (Green, 1999) as decisions made on apparent utilitarian grounds of cost containment seem to have the value of reduced access to, rather than improvement of, clinical services (Thompson et al., 1992). The dilemma faced by psychiatrists, and physicians in general, is to reconcile the needs of the patient with that of the society. Such considerations often bring the physician into conflict with the rest of society (Levinsky, 1984). The notion of a tension between psychiatrists' obligations to their patients and to third parties is protean and has been considered in terms of the so-called dual role dilemma in psychiatric ethics (Robertson & Walter, 2008).

On the 'flip side' of this argument are the ethical responsibilities faced by psychiatrists in resource allocation. Although the procurement and protection of access to limited health care resources is one issue, the alternative is the need for some form of financial responsibility. Much of the cost of health care is decided at the individual clinical level; although exercising fiscal responsibility should not occur with the obscene goal of aiding health maintenance organizations divert health dollars from the clinical setting to corporate profits, the psychiatrist does arguably have ethical obligations to spend mental health dollars wisely (Singh, Hawthorne, & Vos, 2001). One of the problems associated with this obligation is that of quantification. The international standard measures of utility in regard to health care is the Disability Adjusted Life Year (DALY; Murray & Lopez, 1996) and the Quality Adjusted Life Year (QALY; (Williams, 1988), despite the fact that these are insensitive measures when applied to psychiatric disorders (Chisholm, Healy, & Knapp, 1997).

The social contract may fail and lead to social injustice when there is a failure of the sovereign to maintain law and order. This breakdown of law and order may occur as a consequence of some calamity occurring in the state, such as natural disaster or foreign invasion, or when the sovereign perpetrates oppressive violence against its citizens. These circumstances have been seen in totalitarian regimes, where widespread persecution by the state occurs. A vivid example of this was the human rights violations witnessed in Argentina during the period of the military dictatorship that ended in 1982, documented in the CONADEP report (1984). In other circumstances, the sovereign may fail to provide the benefits of the social contract to members of a society who may be part of a persecuted or neglected minority. These groups may be denied the benefits of the social contract as a result of institutionalized racism or on political grounds. Many 'decent' members of the international community, themselves signatories to international covenants of human rights, are capable of such social injustice.

In these circumstances, the ethical remit of psychiatrists in regard to social justice may extend beyond advocacy for those with established mental illness to all those who are disadvantaged and at risk of developing mental illness.

The mental health consequences of politicized violence or denial of the benefits of the social contract arguably represents an area of ethical responsibility for psychiatrists. Moreover, psychiatrists may have ethical responsibilities in the process of restorative justice, in which communities rebuild after such failures of the social contract.

Psychiatrists who live in totalitarian regimes have often been persecuted as a group, or for individual actions or beliefs. Individual psychiatrists 'disappeared' in Argentina under the dictatorship simply for treating survivors of the regime's torture and imprisonment practices (Knudson, 1997). In other circumstances, such as in the former Union of Soviet Socialist Republics, psychiatrists have been complicit in persecution of citizens of a totalitarian regime, often confecting politically based diagnoses as justifications for imprisonment (Bloch & Reddaway, 1983).

In modern Australia, psychiatrists face a particular ethical dilemma, which is an exemplar of the problem of the abuse of human rights in otherwise stable and liberal societies. The policy of recent Australian Federal governments has been to enact a draconian approach towards refugees, who arrive 'unlawfully' in Australian territory. Part of this process involves the mandatory detention of all 'unauthorized illegal entrants', including women and children, in privately operated 'detention centres' (Silove, 2002; Steel & Silove, 2004). Children detained in these settings have been exposed to suicide attempts and self-injurious behaviour by other refugees, compounding their experience of the trauma of the regimes they fled and the perilous voyages made to escape (Steel & Silove, 2001). Given the deleterious consequences of such treatment (Steel, et al., 2006), it is clear that this represents an instance of the sovereign of a nation violating its obligations under the social contract. Although such propositions can be obscured by debates over a nation's/state's rights to sovereignty over territory and the status of unlawful entrants under the social contract, the situation faced by psychiatrists in Australia is, quite simply, the perpetration of the abuse of human rights by the state with whom they exist in a contractual professional relationship. Australian psychiatrists face the ethical dilemma of abiding by the reprehensible policy of their society, manifest in the actions of the popularly elected government or risk politicizing the profession by speaking out against harmful actions by a popularly elected government (Dudley et al., 2004). Such decisions often invoke the political and moral views of individual psychiatrists resulting in divisions within the profession.

Conclusion

Throughout this chapter we have advanced the view that professional psychiatric ethics is best considered in light of social contract theory. We do not endorse the view that such an approach represents a comprehensive account of psychiatric ethics, as many other approaches to the field provide compelling bases of ethical psychiatric practice. Our argument for the contractarian approach to professional psychiatric ethics has the instrumental value of enabling psychiatrists to consider the quandaries they face in their work in the context of a network of relationships between the psychiatrist, the patient, social institutions, and other organs of community. Psychiatric and indeed medical practice now exists as a social good and therefore many more voices are present in the complex discourse of psychiatry. Our argument for the social contract approach to professional psychiatric ethics, and the structural problems such an approach has in the setting of mental illness, aspires to provide a means by which psychiatrists and their professional bodies can be positioned in relation to such a complex discourse.

References

(1978). Declaration of Hawaii. *Journal of Medical Ethics*, **4**, 71–73.

(1984). *Nunca Más (Never Again)* – Report of CONADEP (National Commission on the Disappearance of Persons) – 1984. Retrieved 31 March 2007 from http://www.nuncamas.org/english/library/nevagain/nevagain_001.htm.

(1993). *Oxford English Dictionary* (2nd ed). Oxford: Clarendon Press.

(1997). World Psychiatric Association Approves Declaration of Madrid (25 August 1996). *International Digest of Health Legislation*, **48**, 240–242.

ABIM Foundation, ACP-ASIM Foundation & EFIM (2002). Medical Professionalism in the New Millennium: A Physician Charter *Annals of Internal Medicine*, **136**, 243–246.

Angell, M. (2009). Drug companies & doctors: A story of corruption. *New York Review of Books*, **56**.

Appelbaum, P. (2005). Dangerous severe personality disorders: England's experiment in using psychiatry for public protection. *Psychiatric Services*, **56**, 397–399.

Bloch, S., & Reddaway, P. (1983). *Soviet Psychiatric Abuse*. London: Gollancz.

Borry, P., Schotsmans, P., & Dierickx, K. (2008). The origin and emergence of empirical ethics. In E. E. i. Psychiatry, G. Widdershoven, J. McMillan, et al. (Eds), *Empirical Ethics in Psychiatry* (pp. 37–50). Oxford: Oxford University Press.

Butler, T., Andrews, G., Allnutt, S., et al, (2006). Mental disorders in Australian prisoners: A comparison with a community sample. *Australian and New Zealand Journal of Psychiatry*, **40**, 272–276.

California. Supreme Court., (1973). Tarasoff v. Regents of the University of California. 6 Jul 1973. *West's California Report*, **108**, 878–901.

Chisholm, D., Healy, A., & Knapp, M. (1997). QALYs and mental health care. *Social Psychiatry and Psychiatric Epidemiology*, **32**, 68–75.

Clouser, K. (1970). What is medical ethics? *Annals of Internal Medicine*, **80**.

Clouser, K. (1995). Common morality as an alternative to principlism. *Kennedy Institute of Ethics Journal*, **5**, 219–236.

Clouser, K., & Gert, B. (1990). A critique of principlism. *Journal of Medicine and Philosophy*, **15**, 219–236

Clouser, K. D. (1973). Some things medical ethics is not. *JAMA*, **223**, 787–789.

Coleborne, E. (2003). Introduction: Deinstitutionalisation in Australia and New Zealand *Health & History*, **5**(2), 1–16.

Cruess, R., & Cruess, S. (1997). Teaching medicine as a profession in the service of healing. *Academic Medicine*, **72**, 941–952.

Cruess, S., Johnston, S., & Cruess, R. (2002). Professionalism for medicine: Opportunities and obligations. *Medical Journal of Australia*, **177**, 208–211.

Daniels, N. (1995). *Just Health Care*. Cambridge: Cambridge University Press.

Dax, E. (1981). Crimes, follies and misfortunes in the history of Australasian psychiatry. *Australian and New Zealand Journal of Psychiatry*, **15**, 257–263.

Dhanda, A., & Narayah, T. (2007). Mental health and human rights. *The Lancet*, **370**, 1197–1198.

Dudley, M., Jureidini, J., Mares, S., et al. (2004). In protest. *Australian and New Zealand Journal of Psychiatry*, **38**, 978–979.

Dyer, A. (1988). *Ethics and Psychiatry: Toward a Professional Definition*. New York: American Psychiatric Press.

Engel, G. (1977). The need for a new medical model: a challenge for biomedicine. *Science*, **196**, 129–136.

Engel, G. (1980). The clinical application of the biopsychosocial model. *American Journal of Psychiatry*, **137**, 535–544.

Engelhardt, H. (1996). *The Foundations of Bioethics* (2nd ed). New York: Oxford University Press.

Foucault, M. (1965). *Madness and Civilization R. Howard (trans)*. New York: Pantheon.

Fullinwider, R. (1996). Professional codes and moral understanding. In M. Coady, & S. Bloch (Eds), *Codes of Ethics and the Professions* (pp. 72–87). Melbourne: Melbourne University Press.

Gert, B. (1998). *Morality: Its Nature and Justification*. New York: Oxford University Press.

Gert, B. (2004). *Common Morality: Deciding What to Do*. New York: Oxford University Press.

Ghaemi, N. (2003). *The Concepts of Psychiatry – A Pluralistic Approach to Mind and Mental Illness*. Baltimore: Johns Hopkins University Press.

Green, S. (1999). The ethics of managed mental health care. In S. Bloch, P. Chodoff, & S. Green (Eds), *Psychiatric Ethics* (3rd ed) (pp. 401–21). New York: Oxford University Press.

Green, S. (2008). Ethics and the pharmaceutical industry. *Australasian Psychiatry*, **16**, 158–165.

Green, S., & Bloch, S. (2001). Working in a flawed mental health care system: An ethical challenge. *American Journal Psychiatry*, **158**, 1378–1383.

Healy, D. (1997). *The Antidepressant Era*. Cambridge, MA: Harvard University Press.

Healy, D. (2004). *Let Them Eat Prozac: The Unhealthy Relationship between the Pharmaceutical Industry and Depression*. New York: New York University Press.

Healy, D., & Thase, M. E. (2003). Is academic psychiatry for sale? *British Journal of Psychiatry*, **182**, 388–390.

Herrman, H., & Swartz, L. (2007). Promotion of mental health in poorly resourced countries. *The Lancet,* **370**, 1195–1197

Hobbes, T. (ed). (1651/1985). *Leviathan.* London: Penguin.

Jones, E., & Mendell, L. (1999). Assessing the decade of the brain. *Science* **284**, 739.

Kirk, K., & Kutchins, H. (1997). *Making Us Crazy: The Psychiatric Bible and the Creation of Mental Disorders.* New York: Free Press.

Kirk, S., & Kutchins, H. (1992). *The Selling of the DSM: The Rhetoric of Science in Psychiatry.* New York: Aldine de Gruyer.

Knudson, J. (1997). Veil of silence – the Argentine press and the dirty war. *Latin American Perspectives,* **24**, 93–112.

Levinsky, N. (1984). The doctor's master. *New England Journal of Medicine,* **314**, 1573–1575.

Lewis, M. (1988). *Managing Madness: Psychiatry and Society in Australia 1788–1980,.* Canberra: Australian Government Publishing Service.

Mental Health Council of Australia. (2005). Not for Service: Experiences of Injustice and Despair in Mental Health Care in Australia. Retrieved 10 June 2008 from http://www.mhca.org.au.

Murray, C., & Lopez, A. (1996). *The Global Burden of Disease: A Comprehensive Assessment of Mortality and Disability from Diseases, Injuries, and Risk Factors in 1990 and Projected to 2020.* Washington DC Harvard School of Public Health on Behalf of the World Health Organization and the World Bank.

Nussbaum, M. (1999). *Sex and Social Justice.* New York: Oxford University Press.

Nussbaum, M. (2006). *Frontiers of Justice.* Cambridge, MA: Bellknap.

Pellegrino, E. (1993). The metamorphosis of medical ethics. *Journal of the American Medical Association,* **269**, 1158–1162.

Pellegrino, E. (1999). Professional medical associations: Ethical and practical guidelines. *JAMA,* **282**, 984–986.

Percival, T. (1985). *Codes of Institutes and Precepts Adapted to the Professional Conduct of Physicians and Surgeons.* Birmingham, AL: Classics of Medicine Library.

Plotkin, M. (2001). *Freud in the Pampas.* Stanford: Stanford University Press

Rawls, J. (1971). *A Theory of Justice.* Cambridge, MA: The Bellknap Press.

Rawls, J. (1993). *Political Liberalism.* New York: Columbia University Press.

Rawls, J. (2001). *Justice as Fairness: A Restatement.* Cambridge, MA: Harvard University Press.

Ridenour, N. (1961). *Mental Health in the United States. A Fifty-Year History.* Cambridge, MA: Harvard University Press.

Robertson, M., Kerridge, I., & Walter, G. (2009). Ethnomethodological study of the values of Australian psychiatrists: towards an empirically derived RANZCP Code of Ethics. *Australian and New Zealand Journal of Psychiatry,* **43**, 409–419.

Robertson, M., & Walter, G. (2007). Overview of psychiatric ethics VI: Newer approaches to the field. *Australasian Psychiatry* **15**, 411–416.

Robertson, M., & Walter, G. (2008). The many faces of the dual-role dilemma in psychiatric ethics. *Australian and New Zealand Journal of Psychiatry* **42**, 228–235.

Ross, W. (1939). *The Foundation of Ethics.* Oxford: Clarendon Press.

Sabin, J., & Daniels, N. (1994). Determining 'medical necessity' in mental health practice. *Hastings Center Report*, **24**, 5–13.

Sen, A. (1993). Capability and well-being. In M. Nussbaum, & A. Sen (Eds), *The Quality of Life* (pp. 30–53). Oxford: The Clarendon Press.

Silove, D. (2002). The asylum debacle in Australia: A challenge for psychiatry. *Australian and New Zealand Journal of Psychiatry*, **36**, 290–296.

Singh, B., Hawthorne, G., & Vos, T. (2001). The role of economic evaluation in mental health care. *Australian and New Zealand Journal of Psychiatry*, **35**, 104–117.

Steel, Z., & Silove, D. (2001). The mental health implications of detaining asylum seekers. *Medical Journal of Australia*, **175**, 596–599.

Steel, Z., & Silove, D. (2004). Science and the common good: indefinite, non-reviewable mandatory detention of asylum seekers and the research imperative. *Monash Bioethics Review*, **23**, 93–103.

Steel, Z., Silove, D., Brooks, R., et al. (2006). Impact of immigration detention and temporary protection on the mental health of refugees. *British Journal of Psychiatry*, **188**, 58–64.

Thompson, J., Burns, B., Goldman, H., et al. (1992). Initial level of care and clinical status in a managed mental health care program. *Hospital and Community Psychiatry*, **43**, 599–603.

Wazana, A., & Primeau, F. (2002). Ethical considerations in the relationship between physicians and the pharmaceutical industry. *Psychiatric Clinics of North America* **25**, 647–663.

Welsh, S., & Deahl, M. (2002). Modern psychiatric ethics. *The Lancet*, **359**, 253–255.

White, P., & Whiteford, H. (2006). Prisons: Mental health institutions of te 21st century? *Medical Journal of Australia*, **185**, 302–303.

Williams, A. (1988). Ethics and efficiency in the provision of health care. In J. Bell, & S. Mendus (Eds), *Philosophy and Medical Welfare* (pp. 111–126). New York: Cambridge University Press.

Williams, B. (1972). Relativism. In *Morality: An Introduction to Ethics* (pp. 34–39). Cambridge: Oxford University Press.

Wong, D. (1991). Relativism. In P. Singer (Ed), *A Companion to Ethics* (pp. 442–449). Oxford: Blackwell.

WPA (1996). World Psychiatric Association – Madrid Declaration on Ethical Standards for Psychiatric Practice. Retrieved 23 Nov 2007 from http://www.wpanet.org/generalinfo/ethic1.html.

Chapter 18

Psychiatry's contract: where next?

Dinesh Bhugra and Amit Malik

The relationship between medicine as a profession and society is interdependent and by and large mutually beneficial, even though at times this relationship can be fractious. Medicine's contract with society has been written about by Sylvia Cruess (2006), and the implicit nature of the contract is generally evident. However, psychiatry's position in society and its role is perhaps more controlling of abnormal behaviour and yet possibly more uncertain and ambiguous. In many countries psychiatrists are seen as agents of the state and not as caring health professionals. Psychiatry as a discipline is also shadowed by its reputation and past indiscretions.

Perhaps more than other medical disciplines, as psychiatrists we are influenced by society's expectations. Society defines abnormality and deviance and we as clinicians often have to deal with this no matter how unpalatable it might be. A classic example is that of the removal of homosexuality from the *Diagnostic and Statistical Manual* in the 1970s when, by virtue of its removal, millions of 'mentally ill' people were cured outright. On the one hand, it is the demedicalization of normal human behaviour that psychiatrists lead on and believe in and, on the other, the dangers of medicalizing normal human emotions and responses lead psychiatrists to reposition ourselves. Inherent within such positioning are societal expectations. In the United Kingdom a few years ago, politicians decided to introduce the concept of Dangerous Severe Personality Disorder, much against the advice and indeed the protests of the psychiatric profession. The challenge under such circumstances is for psychiatrists to believe in their professionalism, to protect patients, and to advocate for them.

The clinical practice of psychiatry cannot be seen in isolation from society and culture. The clinical services provided have to be funded by society, which in return expects certain standards of care and health services delivery. Society expects that as a profession we practise to the highest possible clinical standards and meet with their expectations. It is a process where society controls the purse strings and expectations, but professional standards and training are controlled by the profession. In understanding of such a contract, it is the expectations of patients and their families, the public, the media, politicians, policymakers, the third sector, and other stakeholders, which then become important. In addition, the expectations of respect, autonomy, access to knowledge and resources, freedom to practise self-regulation, and financial rewards are some of things that psychiatrists expect in return. In some ways, this is no different from those expected by other doctors. As members of society, psychiatrists need to be more active in discussing with and informing society about psychiatric disorders, stigma, and risk management related to psychiatric disorders.

Professionalism includes a technical scientific knowledge base, altruism, commitment to professional competence, honesty, probity, awareness of just distribution of finite resources, maintenance of trust, and self-regulation. At its core, medical professionalism contains the principles of primacy of patient welfare, linked with patient autonomy and social justice (American College of Physicians, 2002). Embedded within these principles are components of improving both cost-effectiveness and access to good quality care. Society expects that members of the profession will keep their knowledge up to date and not only maintain but also expand their skills base. Profession is a socially based activity (Racy, 1990). Within such activities, the core is the patient–psychiatrist interaction sanctioned by society. Ethical and moral values are imparted by the society and the culture within which psychiatrists practise. Regulatory bodies for the profession ensure that this actually happens. Recent perceived threats to professionalism and the profession come from many sources (Bhugra, 2008). Increasing patient knowledge and ease of access to such knowledge through the Internet and other sources means that the power differential that previously existed between doctors and patients is beginning to disappear. Patients often appear in the clinic with printouts of their conditions and side-effects of drugs, and are able to ask more penetrating questions. Consequently, the old-fashioned patriarchal model is giving way to a more collaborative approach between the patient and the psychiatrist. In addition, the changing political climate, with more prescriptive policies and increased regulation, has affected the psychiatrist's autonomy.

As Cruess (2006) reminds us, medicine's contract with society emerged about 300 years ago. With increasingly technical medicine and newer developments such as pharmacogenomics, the ethical landscape is beginning to shift. Medical and psychiatric scandals in the United Kingdom and the United States in the last 30 years or so have shaken the public's trust in doctors, even though doctors remain the most trusted profession compared to others. Society, as Cruess (2006) notes, expects the services of a competent, caring, altruistic healer, with moral and ethical values. Changes in funding in the United States and elsewhere will bring a different set of expectations by society of the profession.

Furthermore, the economic downturn in large parts of the world is likely to concentrate on demands for cost-effective but efficacious health care delivery.

Patients expect collaboration, shared information, and competence from their psychiatrists. The public in general expects the same, as do employers. Thus there are several common strands in these expectations with which the profession can work to re-evaluate its contract with society.

Apart from the economic downturn, other challenges include an increasingly technical specialty, fiduciary responsibility, and increasing demand with shrinking resources. Changing expectations of allowing the profession to self-regulate are emerging. There are possibilities of other professions being allowed to prescribe medication, which will influence the role of doctors. In addition, a target-driven health care delivery rather than an outcome-based one; increasing consumerism where medicine (psychiatry in this case) is seen as a business and a product which people can buy as in a supermarket, and internalized demoralization of the profession are all challenges that need to be overcome using a number of strategies. What is vital is public education, the reduction of stigma towards mental illness and the mentally ill, advocacy and working with patients and families, making efficient use of evidence-based treatments, in addition to instilling professional values in undergraduate students and with regular updates and continued professional developments. Learning through mentoring, clinical practice, observation, and other methods are all important steps. The professional values of the profession are important, as are the perceived values held by society. Courses in ethics and other related aspects of professional values can provide a springboard for personal growth and development. The primacy of patient welfare and advocacy for the patients, their carers and families remain paramount in delivery of services. Taking a scientific and evidence base allows psychiatrists to be aware of their responsibilities in ensuring high-quality services which are physically, geographically, and emotionally accessible. Emotional intelligence is important in clinical settings, but clinical knowledge and scientific basis of psychiatry can only strengthen our relationship and contract with society.

References

American College of Physicians. (2002). Medical professionalism in the new millennium: A physician's charter. *Annals of Internal Medicine,* **136,** 243–246.

Bhugra, D. (2008). Professionalism and psychiatry: The profession speaks. *Acta Psychiatrica Scandinavica,* **118,** 327–329.

Cruess, S. R. (2006). Professionalism and medicine's contract with society. *Clinical Orthopaedics and Related Research,* **449,** 170–176.

Racy, J. (1990). Professionalism: Sane and insane. *Journal of Clinical Psychiatry,* **51,** 138–140.

Index

academic training 79; *see also* training
Academy of Medical Royal Colleges 191–2
accountability 27–8, 199, 216
accreditation 150–1, *153*, 154–5, 157, 158, 189
adaptation 213; *see also* changing health care environments
advocacy 223, 232–3, *233*, 234, 241, 243
affect *90*, 90
affirmation 168
age discrimination 47–8
alienism 228
altruism 4
 professional 29–31, 36, 104
 psychiatry trainees 65–6
 and self-regulation 110, 111
 and social contracts 136, 137
Alzheimer's disease 18
Alzheimer, Kraepelin, Wernicke 11
American Medical Association (AMA) 43, 129, 138
American Psychiatric Association 11, 43, 50, 51, 151, 230–1, 241
antidepressants 230
anti-psychiatry movement 171
anxiety 95
appraisal, revalidation 184–6
apprenticeship model 77, 183
Argentina 229, 234, 235
arrogance 199–200
art of medicine 113
Ashley, Lord 13–14
assertive citizens 212
assessment procedures 177, 186–7
Association of Medical Officers of Asylums for the Insane 11
Association of Superintendents of American Institutions for the Insane 11
asylums, history 11
attachment relationships 90, 92
attitudes, doctors 165
audit 187–8, 190, 215
Australia 229, 235
authority, scepticism towards 103
autonomy 2, 4–5; *see also* self-regulation
 doctor-patient relationship 213
 conflicts of 214, 225
 and ethics 223
 future developments 242

regulatory framework 135
and social contracts 124, 125, 136
training 109

baby P 206
Balint training 66
beaurocracy 2, 27–8, 45
Beers, Clifford 13
benefit/harm ratios 6
Bennett, David 37
best practice 56–7
Bethlem Royal Hospital 11
biological model 84, 90–1, 95–6, 171
biopsychosocial model 91, 221, 228
black and minority ethnic (BME) groups 37, 38–9, 47
blind men and the elephant parable 206
blindfold of justice 227
bonds, professional 25–6
Breaking the Circles of Fear (Sainsbury Trust) 37
Bristol cases 135, 199
British Medical Association (BMA) 128–9
bullying, staff 167
burnout 66, 74
Bush, President George 230
businesses 29–32

Calman reforms 77
Canada 129
Canadian Medical Association (CMA) 129
Canadian Medical Education Directives for Specialists (CanMEDS) 77
Canterbury Tales (Chaucer) 26
capabilities approach 48, 225, 226
capitalism 1–2
cardiovascular surgery, outcome measurement 188, 216
care in the community 15, 66, 74–5, 229–30
Care Quality Commission (CQC) 152
carers 64, 92
case-based discussion 186–7
causation, mental illness 90–1
CBT (cognitive behaviour therapy) 19, 95
challenges
 future 243
 to professionalism 210–11
challenging patients 65–6

changing health care environments 202–3, 209
  challenges to professionalism 210–11
  doctor-patient relationship 214–15
  empowerment of citizens/consumers 212
  empowerment of patients 212–13, 213–14
  ethics, psychiatric 228–31
  future developments 219
  implications 218–19
  involving patients in decision-making 213–14
  new professionalism 219–20
  political empowerment 217–18
  power shifts 211–12
  professionalism 209–10
  quality improvement 215–17
child guidance 18
China 36
chlorpromazine 229
choice 98, 149
  criteria 44, 49–51
  and doctor-patient relationship 92
  lifestyle 219
  NHS agenda 214
Choices websites 154
clinical leadership 67–8, 176; see also leadership
Clinical Negligence Scheme for Trusts 164, 167
clinical practice guidelines see guidelines
codes of conduct 1–2
cognitive behaviour therapy (CBT) 19, 95
collaboration
  patient/doctor 198–9; see also sharing knowledge/information
  professional 55–6
collective good 223
Commission for Health Improvement (Health Care Commission) 152, 167
commissioning reforms, healthcare 173–5
common morality theory 226–8
communication 6, 25
  changing health care environments 218
  collaboration 56
  doctor-patient relationship 165, 214
  and explanatory models 39
  and performance management/regulation 149
  physicians 36, 64, 69
  research issues 53
communist abuse 14
community care 15, 66, 74–5, 229–30
community psychiatry 14, 15, 16–19
complaints/serious incidents 191, 215; see also medical scandals
complementary medicine 67–8
compulsory treatment 73, 80, 89; see also safety
conduct, professional see regulation
confidentiality 26, 161

conflict of interest
  carers 92
  dual role dilemma 231, 233, 241; see also safety, public
  magagerial perspectives 201–2
  medical profession 136
  and social contracts 135–7
  society/mentally ill 226–8
Constitution, NHS 197
consultants, NHS 81–3
consumerist agenda 212, 213, 220, 222, 243
continuing education 51
continuing professional development (CPD) 51, 184, 188–90, 243
continuity, teaching 112
continuity of care 76
contracting and commissioning 150, 161
contracts with society see social contracts
cost-effectiveness 46
counter-transference 94
covenants 124
CPD (continuing professional development) 184, 188–90, 243
crafts 32
crises, psychiatric 53, 76
criteria
  choice 44, 49–51
  efficiency 45–6
  equity 46–8
  evaluative 23–8
  health care quality 148
  professional 23–8, 44
critical psychiatry 171
Critical Psychiatry Network 39
criticism 98
cultural factors 127
customer satisfaction 80; see also consumerist agenda; patients

DALYs (Disability Adjusted Life Years) 234
dangerous severe personality disorder 229, 241
Darzi report 78, 174, 197
debates, psychiatric 54–5
decision-making
  choice criteria 50
  economics of psychiatry 54
  efficiency criteria 45–6
  involving patients 198, 200, 213–14, 218
Declaration of Madrid 230, 232
defensiveness, psychiatry profession 39, 40, 187
definitions
  cost-effectiveness 46
  doctors 9
  efficiency 44
  equity 44
  forensic psychiatry 18

health care 225
professionalism 109
professions 23–8, 221–2
psychiatry 9, 19
regulation/scrutiny/litigation 163
social contracts 124
deinstitutionalization 15
deliberate self-harm (DSH) 96–7
demand-side reforms 173
depression 68, 92, 95, 230
deprofessionalization 81–3
diagnosis 91, 92
Diagnostic and Statistical Manual of Mental Disorders (American Psychiatric Association) 230–1, 241
dialogue, doctor-patient 92
difference, pathologizing 36–7
difficult patients 65–6
Disability Adjusted Life Years (DALYs) 234
disability model 38
discrimination 47–8, 200–1
dismissive attitudes, doctors' 165
distrust *see* trust
diversity, psychiatric 16–19
doctor-patient relationship 1, 98, 165, 242
    changing health care environments 214–15, 217, 218
    partnership 213–14, 218
    and patient choice 92
    and patient engagement 61
    and politics 53
    social contracts 89
    and stakeholder expectations 59–60, *60*, *61*
    training 65
doctors
    conflicts with management 201–2
    definition 9
    mental health 83–4
    perspectives on psychiatry 97
The Doctor's Dilemma (Shaw) 210
Doctors in Society (Royal College of Physicians) 195
dosage guidelines 158, *160*
DSH (deliberate self-harm) 96–7
dual role dilemma 231, 233, 241; *see also* conflicts of interest; safety

Earl of Shaftesbury 13–14
economics 43–4, 55–7, 242–3
    barriers to improvement 51–5
    choice 49–51
    efficiency criteria 44–6
    equity 46–8
    great debates 54–5
    and health care quality 148
    managerial models 96–7
    medication model 95–6
    professional issues 53–4

research issues 52–3, 56
and social contracts 136, 137
and teaching professionalism 74, 103
education *90*, 210; *see also* continuing professional development; training
efficiency 44–6
electro-convulsive therapy (ECT) 154, 157, 158, *159*
emergency work 53, 76
emotion *90*
emotional intelligence 73, *90*, 243
empathy 61–2, 63, 65, 69, 202
employers, expectations 67–9
empowerment 50, *90*, 91; *see also* choice criteria
    citizens/consumers 212
    patients 212–13, 213–14, 228
    political 217–18
    professional issues 53
    quality improvement 215–17
enforced treatment 73, 80, 89; *see also* safety
engagement
    patient 61
    professional *90*
England; *see also* United Kingdom
    performance management/ regulation 152–4
    social contracts 172–8
Enlightenment 219
environment, healthcare 107–8, 149
equity 96
    criteria 46–8, 149
    definition 44
    magagerial perspectives 204–5
    and social contracts 126
    and teaching professionalism 108
    treatment 38
ethics, psychiatric *90*, 221, 235–6, 243; *see also* values
    changing health care environments 228–31
    conflicts of interest, social/psychiatric values 226–8
    justice, social 231–5
    new professionalism 221–4
    professional 24, 26
    and social contracts 224–6, 231, 235–6
    universal standards 16
ethos 210
European Union of Medical Specialties (UEMS) 17
evaluation, teaching professionalism 114–15
evidence-based psychiatry 5–6, 43, *90*, *90*, 243
    debates, psychiatric 55
    medicine/psychiatry 10, 220
    new approaches 41
    research issues 52–3
    United Kingdom 17

expectations 41, 74
  carers 64
  changing health care environments 218
  distrust of mental health system 36–8
  employers 67–9
  legitimate 136
  new approaches to psychiatry 39–40, 41
  and obligations 3–4, 37, 133, *134*
  physician 62
  practice/perception problems 38–9
  public 66–7
  reciprocity 109
  and social contracts 126, *132*, *133*, *134*, 241–2
  stakeholders 59–64, *60*, *61*, 69, 89, 241–3
  stigma of psychiatry 35–6
  therapeutic relationship/health system factors 61–4
  trainees 64–6
experiential learning 105, 109–12
expert patients 198
expert witnesses 167
expertise *90*, 92
explanatory models 5, 38–9
  new approaches 39–40, 41
  and stakeholder expectations 59, 60, 64
extermination of mentally ill 12, 14

faculty development 113–14
families 32, 89, 92
fairness *see* equity
fear of mentally ill 37
feedback appraisal 190–1
flexibility of mind 24–5
forensic psychiatry 18
formal curriculum 108
framework of capabilities, multidisciplinary teams 93–4
France 135
freedom of choice *see* choice
funding psychiatry training 79–80
  futures 138, 241–3

gag laws 133–4
General Medical Council (GMC) 129
  assessment procedures 177
  criticism 163–4
  good doctor framework 78
  Good Medical Practice 196
  revalidation 181. *see also* revalidation
genomics 242
Germany 12, 14, 15, 36
globalization 230–1
good doctor framework 78
Good Doctors' Safer Patients (Chief Medical Officer for England) 182
Good Medical Practice (General Medical Council) 196

Good Psychiatry Practice (Royal College of Psychiatrists) 181, 186
guidelines
  and autonomy 54
  clinical practice 5–6
  dosage 158, *160*
  NICE 158
  performance management/regulation 149
  UK/US 43

handover of patients 76
harm/benefit ratios 6
healer role 83–4, *84–5*, 89, 98, 111
  physicians 64
  and social contracts 127
  and soul 41
health care
  definition 225
  quality challenge 148–9
  and social contracts 133–4
Health Care Commission 152, 167
health insurance 138
hidden curriculum 108
High Quality Care for All (Darzi report) 78, 174, 197
Hippocratic tradition 103, 221, 222, 223
historic treatment of mentally ill 10, 12–13
Hobbes, Thomas 224
holistic treatment 5, 6
homosexuality 241
honesty 64
human rights approach 204–5, 229, 234, 235

identification of unsatisfactory practice 169
ideological models 95
Idiot's Act 18
illegal immigrants 235
implicit bargains 1–4, 5, 6, 124, 125; *see also* social contracts
individuality 25, 54; *see also* autonomy
infantilization of patients 62
informal curriculum 108
information/knowledge 242
  accurate 51
  overload 43, 57
  ownership 32
  partnership 218
  patient 74
  power shifts 211
  sharing 214–15; *see also* collaboration
  systems 175
Inside Outside (Department of Health) 37
insight, physician 84
institutional leadership 67–8; *see also* leadership
institutional support 106–7
International Code of Medical Ethics (World Medical Association) 43–4
internet 242
  debates, psychiatric 54–5

empowerment of patients 213
expert patients 198
impact on psychiatry 51
power shifts 212
and stakeholder expectations 64
investment in healthcare services 175

judgement 195
justice, social
 normal function model 226
 and professional ethics 231–5
 Rawl's theory 126

knowledge *see* information/knowledge

la douceur 10
Laing, R. D. 171
leadership 82, 98, 172, 195, 202
 clinical 67–8, 176
 institutional 67–8
 magagerial perspectives 203–4
 and performance management/
  regulation 149
 and teaching professionalism 107, 198
learning disability 18
legislation 73, 82, 136, 137
levers for improvement 149–51
life unworthy of life 12, 14
lifelong learning 51
lifestyle choices 219
litigation 2, 30, 74, 164; *see also* regulation
Lord Ashley 13–14

Madness and Civilization (Foucault) 36
managed care 233
management
 appraisal 192
 boards 150, 161
 cultures 95
 models 96–7
managerial perspectives 195–8, 206–7
 arrogance 199–200
 changing health care environments 202–3
 conflicts with doctors 201–2
 discrimination 200–1
 duties of a doctor 196
 empathy 202
 equity/human rights 204–5
 leadership 202, 203–4
 moral compass 201
 paternalism 198–9
 respecting patients 200
 systems thinking 206
 transparency/accountability 199
 values 205–6
market economy 49, 50, 125
maximin principles 48
MDTs *see* multidisciplinary teams
meaning of illness 40, 61

medical model 38
media roles 135
medical leadership *see* leadership
Medical Leadership Competency
 Framework 78
medical model 84, 90–1, 95–6, 171; *see also*
 biopsychosocial model
medical profession 130, *131*; *see also*
 professionalism
Medical Research Council (MRC) 79
Medical Revalidation Principles and Next Steps
 (Department of Health) 182
medical scandals 3, 23, 163, 242
 baby P 206
 Bristol cases 135
 complaints/serious incidents 191, 215
 and social contracts 123, 136
medication 38
 dosage guidelines 158, *160*
 model 95–6
 non-medical prescribing 74–5, 243
 and professional ethics 229–30
 and stakeholder expectations 62
medicine
 as service industry 222
 and society 4
*Medicopsychological Association and Royal
 Medicopsychological Association* 11
medieval guilds 1–2
Mental Aftercare Association 13
Mental Health Act 37
mental health paradigm 228
mental hygiene movement 13, 228
mentally ill, history of treatment 10, 12–13
Mid Staffordshire NHS Foundation Trust 200
The MInd that Found Itself (Beers) 13
mindfullness 111
models of care 73, 74–5, 93–4; *see also* care in
 the community
modernizing medical careers (MMC) 77–8
Monitor 152
monopoly, expertise 2, 3, 92, 128, 214
moral/s; *see also* ethics; values
 compass 201
 contracts 124, 125; see also social contracts
 duty 26–7
 high ground 30, 32
 relativism 228
morbidity, mental illness 90
MRC (Medical Research Council) 79
Muller, Hermann Joseph 38
multidisciplinary models 77
multidisciplinary teams (MDTs) 93–5, 97–8
 assessment procedures 177
 framework of capabilities *93–4*
 performance management/
  regulation 147–8
 professional conduct 166–7
multi-source feedback 190–1

National Clinical Assessment Service (NCAS) 164
National Collaborating Centre for Mental Health (NCMH) 17
National Health Service *see* NHS
National Institute for Health and Clinical Excellence *see* NICE
National Institute for Health (NIH) 79
National Institute for Health Research (NIHR) 79
national policy 157
National Service Framework 172, 178
Nazi Germany 12, 14, 15
NCAS (National Clinical Assessment Service) 164
NCMH (National Collaborating Centre for Mental Health) 17
negligence 164; *see also* regulation
negotiation 137–8
new approaches to psychiatry 39–40, 41
New Horizons (Department of Health) 178
new professionalism 109, 219–24
new ways of working (NWW) 74, 82
Next Stage Review 152–3
NHS (National Health Service)
   appraisal 185
   audit 215
   changing health care environments 218
   Constitution 197
   performance management/regulation 152–4
   privatization 1
   reforms, healthcare 172–8
   values 205–6
National Health Service Plan 172
NICE (National Institute for Health and Clinical Excellence)
   choice criteria 50
   efficiency criteria 46
   guidelines 43, 158
   performance management/regulation 152
   quality standards 153, 157
   reforms, healthcare 174
   standards for systems 167
NIH (National Institute for Health) 79
non-clinical practice, appraisal 191–2
non-medical prescribing 74–5, 243
normal function model 226
nostalgic professionalism 109
nurses
   perspectives on psychiatry 97
   survey 67–8
NWW (new ways of working) 74, 82

objectivity 54–5, 56
obligations
   and expectations 3–4, 37, 133, *134*

and privilege 127
and responsibility 124
and social contracts 137
old age psychiatry 18
onion skin model of advocacy 232–3, *233*
out of hours care 76
outcomes
   and doctor-patient relationship 94
   measurement 52–3, 175–6, 188

partnership model 213–14, 218
paternalism 26, 64, 242
   changing health care environments 213, 214
   choice criteria 50
   magagerial perspectives 198–9
patient/s
   centredness 6, 69
   choice *see* choice
   doctor relationship *see* doctor-patient relationship
   empowerment 212–13, 213–14
   expectations *see* expectations
patriarchal model *see* paternalism
patronizing attitudes, doctors' 165
peer pressure 113
peer review 150–1
perception problems, psychiatry 39, 40
performance evaluation 215–16
performance management/regulation 147–8, 161
   England 152–4, *153*
   health care quality challenge 148–9
   improvement mechanisms 156–61
   levers for improvement 149–51
   professional bodies 151
   public reporting 150, 158–61, *159*, *160*
   quality improvement activities 154–6, *156*, 157
   review process 156
personalization 50; *see also* choice criteria
perspectives on psychiatry 95–7
pharmaceutical companies 52–3
   critical psychiatry 171
   medication model 95
   and professional ethics 230
   role in psychiatry 54–5, 56
physician heal thyself 83–4, *84–5*; *see also* doctors
Pinel, Philippe 10
placebo effect 62
policy guidelines *see* guidelines
politics
   and changing health care environments 202–3
   choice criteria 50
   empowerment 217–18

and professional ethics 228–9
and professions 26–7
and psychiatry 14–15, 36
and social contracts 125
Portugal 16
post code lottery 5
post-psychiatry 40
power shifts 211–12, 242
practice problems, psychiatry 38–9, 40
Practitioner Health Programme 169
  preferences *see* choice
prescribing, non-medical 74–5, 243
President George Bush 230
prestige, professional 3, 23, 27, 30
Principles of Medical Ethics (American Medical
  Association) 43
private sector/privatization 1, 133–4, 166
privilege
  and obligations 127
  and rights 109
  self-regulation as 168
  and social contracts 136
probity 166
professional
  bodies 81–3, 137–8, 151
  conduct see regulation
  culture 74
  diversity 16–19
  issues, economic 53–4
professionalism 2, 12–16, 68
  arrogance 199–200
  challenges to 210–11
  changing health care environments 209–10
  definition 12, 13, 109
  discrimination 200–1
  empathy 202
  equity/human rights 204–5
  essence of 242
  failures 10–12, 206
  leadership 202, 203–4
  magagerial perspectives 195, 197
  moral compass 201
  new 109, 219–24
  obstacles *198*; *see also* managerial
    perspectives
  paternalism 198–9
  psychiatry trainees 65–6
  respecting patients 200
  and revalidation 183–4, 192
  seven Es of *90*
  teaching *see* training
  threats to 4–5
  transparency/accountability 199
  values 205–6
professions
  businesses 29–32
  definitions/evaluative criteria 23–8 221–2

and ethics 23
other occupations 28
and politics 26–7
trades/crafts 32
proximate causes of mental illness 91
psychiatry 9–10, 19; *see also* doctors;
    professionalism; training
  definition 9, 19
  diversity 16–19
  early development/failures 10–12
  evidence-based psychiatry 5–6
  great debates 54–5
  new approaches to psychiatry 39–40, 41
  patient-based psychiatry 6, 69
  practice/perception problems 38–9
  stigma 35–6
Psychiatry for the Person (World Psychiatric
    Association) 39–40
psychoanalysis 19
psychologists 97
psychology 35
psychosocial factors 6
psychotherapy 19, 83–4
public expectations 66–7
public reporting 150, 158–61, *159*, *160*,
    215–16
punitive psychiatry 12, 14, 36

qualities needed for psychiatry 165, 222
quality
  criteria 49
  health care systems 148–9
  improvements 154, 215–17
  of life 52, 54, 234
  observatory 154
  standards 153, 157
Quality Adjusted Life Years (QALYs) 234
Quality Improvement Network for Inpatient
    Child and Adolescent Mental Health
    Services 154
quantitative measurement instruments 61, 96

racism 37
Rawls, John 225
recertification 182–3
reciprocity 109, 127, 130
recovery model 92
recruitment, psychiatrists 74, 80–1, *81*; *see
    also* selection
reductionism 38, 54, 95
reflective practice
  multidisciplinary teams 94
  psychiatry trainees 65, 66
  teaching professionalism 73, 105, 109–12
reforms
  healthcare 138–9, 172–8
  training 77–9

refugees 235
registration 210
regulation 166, 169; *see also* performance management/regulation; self-regulation
    concerns 163–4
    definitions 163
    doctors as individuals 165–6
    doctors as part of a system 166–7
    frameworks 135, 150
    lay involvement 216
    patient problems with doctors 164–5
    professionalism 168–9, 210
    and social contracts 135
    standards for systems 167
    reil 10
relationships
    professional 25–6
    with patients *see* doctor-patient relationship
relicensing 184–5
religion 16
research
    appraisal 192
    and economics 52–3, 56
    issues 78, *90*
Resident Wellness Programmes 83
resilience, emotional 90
resource allocation 234
respect
    for doctors 64, 183
    for patients 200
responsibility 243
    levels 5
    medical 75
    and obligations 124
    patient 219
    and rights 214
    and teaching professionalism 107
revalidation 181–3, 193
    appraisal 184–6
    audit 187–8, 190
    case-based discussion 186–7
    changing health care environments 215, 216
    complaints/serious incidents 191
    continuing professional development 188–90
    dealing with areas of concern 192–3
    multi-source feedback 190–1
    non-clinical practice 191–2
    outcome measurement 188
    and professionalism 183–4, 192
rights
    approach 204–5, 229, 234, 235
    and privileges 109
    and responsibilities 214
risk aversion 66, 73
rivalry, multidisciplinary teams 93–4
role models, professional 103–5, 112–13

Royal Australian and New Zealand College of Psychiatrists 151
Royal College of Physicians 11, 27, 195
Royal College of Psychiatrists 18, 19, 77, 129
    accreditation schemes *153*, 154, 157, 158
    appraisal 185, 186, 187
    audit 188
    continuing professional development 190
    history 11, 12
    new approaches to psychiatry 39–40
    outcome measurement 188
    performance management/regulation 151
    quality improvement standards 154–6, *156*, 157, 158, *159*, 184
    revalidation aims 182–3
    website 10
Russia 36, 229, 230, 235

safety, public
    dual role dilemma 231, 233, 241; *see also* conflicts of interest
    and mental illness 224–5; *see also* compulsory treatment
scandals, medical *see* medical scandals
scapegoating 55
schizophrenia 67, 229–30
scientific basis of treatment *see* evidence-based psychiatry
second class citizens 232
sectioning patients 73; *see also* compulsory treatment; safety
selection, doctors 165; *see also* recruitment
self-awareness, physician 83–4
self-interest 29, 224
self-knowledge, physician 83–4
self-regulation 83, 184; *see also* autonomy
    changing health care environments 216
    and ethics 223
    evaluation 115
    and expectations 243
    and medical scandals 135
    professional 3–4, 27–8
    and professional conduct 168
    and self-interest 224
    and social contracts 123–4, 136, 137
    and teaching professionalism 104, 109, 110, 111
sensitivity, physician 84
sharing knowledge/information 214–15; *see also* collaboration
Shaw, George Bernard 210
Shipman Inquiry 181
Smith, Adam 29, 31, 49
Smith, Dame Janet 181
social contracts 1–4, 89, 97–8, 123–4, 138–9
    changing health care environments 219
    definition 124
    doctor-patient relationship/patient choice 92

and economics of psychiatry 51, 56–7
English perspective 172–8
and ethics 224–6, 231, 235–6
evolution 127–30
expectations 126, *132*, *133*, *134*, 241–2
external influences 133–5
framework of capabilities *93–4*
future requirements 138, 241–3
health care system/private sector 133–4
media role 135
nature of clinical psychiatry 89–91
origins/evolution of 124–7
perspectives on psychiatry 95–7
professional bodies/negotiation 137–8
professional status of medicine 109
regulatory framework 135
stakeholders 130–3, *131*
strains/pressures on 135–7
systemic/multidisciplinary issues 92–5, 97–8
training and professionalism 73, 109
social exclusion/inclusion 10, 13–14, 38, 48
social workers, perspectives on psychiatry 97
socialization of doctors 106, 110, 116
society 1–4, 131, *131*
  conflicts of interest 226–8
socio-demographic factors 63
sophisticated moral relativism 228
soul, healing 41
Soviet Union 14
specialization 82, 128
spirituality 16, 89, 91, 98
splitting, multidisciplinary teams 94
St Mary Bethlehem 11
stakeholders
  expectations *see* expectations
  and social contracts 128, 130–3, *131*
standards 3, 241
  implementation 157
  NICE 153, 157
  performance management/regulation 150
  professional 31, 68
  Royal College of Psychiatrists 154–6, *156*, 157, 158, *159*, 184
  systems 167
  training 77
  universal 16
status, professional 3, 23, 27, 30
stereotyping 25
sterilization, compulsory 14
stigma of mental illness 242, 243
  and choice 49
  and equity 48
  and performance management/regulation 149
  physician 35–6, 84
  and professional ethics 232
  public expectations 66
  reducing 64

Strategic Health Authorities 174
stress, doctors 83–4, 103, 167
Sufi parable, blind men and the elephant 206
suicide, physician 83
summative assessment 115
supply-side reforms 173
system management reforms 173
systems thinking, magagerial perspectives 206
Szasz, Thomas 171

target setting 176
teaching *see* training
teamwork 69, 77
terrorists, interrogation 16
therapeutic relationship *see* doctor-patient relationship
therapy, for physicians 83–4
timescales, identification of unsatisfactory practice 169
totalitarian regimes 36, 229, 230, 235
together 13
trade, medicine as 32, 183, 184
trade-offs 54
training, professional 73–4, 84–5, 98, 103–4, 116, 243
  academic 79
  appraisal 192
  assessment 166
  continuity 112
  environment 107–8
  evaluation 114–15
  experiential learning/reflection 109–12
  faculty development 113–14
  funding 79–80
  incremental approach 116
  institutional support 106–7
  leadership skills 107, 198, 204
  models of care 73, 74–5
  physician heal thyself 83–4, *84*–5
  principles 106
  professional bodies/deprofessionalization 81–3
  recruitment challenges/shortfall 74, 80–1, *81*
  reforms, training 77–9
  role modelling 112–13
  stakeholder expectations 64–6
  theoretical background 104–6, 108–9, 115
  trainees, psychiatry 64–6
  working hours 75–6
transactional reforms 173
transparency 183
  appraisal 185
  magagerial perspectives 199
  outcome measurement 188
  power shifts 212
  and professional conduct 168
treatment of mentally ill, history 10, 12–13

trust 128, 183, 218, 242
  mental health system 36–8
  new approaches to psychiatry 41
  patient-physician 5, 164–5
  and social contracts 136
Trust, Assurance and Safety (HMSO) 182

UEMS (European Union of Medical Specialties) 17
United Kingdom
  academic training 79
  Bristol cases 135
  British Medical Association 128–9
  community psychiatry 15–16
  England 152–4
  guidelines 43
  psychiatry 17–19
  Royal College of Psychiatrists 77
  training 77–8
United States of America
  guidelines 43
  managed care 233
  National Institute for Health 79
  National Institute for Health Research 79
USSR 36, 229, 230, 235

values 205–6, 243
  conflicts of interest 226–8
  evaluation 115
  patient 91
  professional 24, 69, 223, 243
  societal 19
  and stakeholder expectations 62
  and teaching professionalism 111
values-based practice 40
virtues, professional 222, 223
vocation, medicine as 165, 183, 184
vulgar moral relativism 228
The Wealth of Nations (Smith) 29, 31

website, Royal College of Psychiatrists 10
welfare model 226
whistle-blowing 31
whole systems thinking 206
wisdom 195
working hours 75–6
workplace-based assessments 186–7
World Class Commissioning 175
World Medical Association (WMA) 43–4, 50
World Psychiatric Association 16, 39–40, 230

York Retreat 16

Zen and the Art of Motorcycle Maintenance (Pirsig) 32